A FAIR ISLE NURSE

A
FAIR
ISLE
NURSE

Mona McAlpine

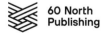

60 North
Publishing

60 North Publishing
7 Mounthooly Street
Lerwick
Shetland
ZE1 0BJ

www.60northpublishing.com

First published in Great Britain in 2022 by 60 North Publishing

'Fair Isle Then' colour photography by Nick Dymond
'Fair Isle Now' photography copyright © Susan Molloy

A catalogue record for this book is available from the British Library

ISBN 978-1-80068-764-6

Cover and layout by Left Design

Printed and bound in the UK by Taylor Brothers Bristol.

For more information visit www.60northpublishing.com

ACKNOWLEDGEMENTS

Misa Hay, Tom Morton, Jenny Henry,
Davie Gardner, Richard Beynon,
Jo-Anne Richards, Trish Urquhart.

Close friends and family.

Wonderful, kind and generous people
of Fair Isle and Shetland.

My two supportive sons
Iain McAlpine and Sven McAlpine.

CHAPTER 1

'I suppose it's a bit late in the day to turn back, Dad? I confess I'm feeling a bit out of my depth and nervous. In fact, I'm terrified.'

The arm that has comforted me all my life is now around my shoulders. 'Now lass, enough of that. Where's that backbone I'm so proud of? You're going to be just fine, believe you me. All those years of training and now you're going to get a chance to show what you're made of.'

Dad takes his eyes off the road for a moment to give me a wink. He's my champion and, holding back the tears, I give him a tentative smile.

This long and winding road runs 25 miles from our home in Whiteness, on the Shetland mainland, to Grutness on the south tip of the island, where I am to board the *Good Shepherd II*, the mail boat that will take me to my new post in Fair Isle. I'm not sure if I want this road to go on forever, or for my journey to begin quickly so that I can get on with the next phase of my life.

I look out the window at the familiar scenery rushing by. It's August, the month when the bonnie purple heather is in full bloom. Peats that have been cut from the hills are all stacked and ready to be bagged. They seem to be waiting patiently for someone to come and take them home. Those trusty peats will keep many a Shetland family warm throughout winter.

I try hard to swallow the lump in my throat. I look at my dear dad with pride and the deep admiration only a daughter can give her loving father, and I know this is a moment I will treasure and hold with me forever.

We race along the narrow road, far too fast, of course, but dad is a competent driver and I have always felt safe in his car. A warm feeling of nostalgia takes over and I ease briefly into dreamlike state.

I am wakened from my semi-slumber when we pull up to an old stone building near the harbour. We are greeted with a hearty 'Hello' from Christine, who runs the Grutness post office. There's no sign yet of the *Good Shepherd*.

I feel light-headed and somewhat nauseous at the prospect that lies before me. Dad looks at me knowingly, and gives Christine a smile as he takes the luggage from the boot of the car. The *Good Shepherd* berths at the pier below her house and I feel sure she is well used to white-faced passengers.

Her cheery smile shakes me out of my mood of nervous apprehension. 'You're going to be the new nurse in Fair Isle, good for you. It'll be a great experience, I'm sure you'll love it.'

Christine certainly knows how to cheer me up. Her sister Agnes is married to my brother, so this feels oddly like a family reunion rather than a wrenching farewell.

'I've been telling her that, Christine,' says dad, 'not that I have ever been to Fair Isle, but I hear it's a bonnie place with a lot going for it. Scenery and wildlife and the bird observatory – she'll be just fine.'

'Oh, for sure,' says Christine, busily sorting out the mail. Mail bags and trays of letters litter the counter. I can even see one bag with a 'Fair Isle' label attached. 'I love Fair Isle,' Christine lifts her expressive eyebrows, 'I'm certainly not fond of the journey, but once there, I'm sometimes tempted to stay.'

'Hear that, Mona,' dad is smiling broadly. 'We'll maybe lose you to the isle! Don't get too fond of it.'

'The *Shepherd* will be here in a peerie start,' says Christine. 'Maybe in half an hour.'

"Peerie" must be the most famous word in the Shetland dialect. It means small. Peerie start means in a short time. Peerie wife, small girl. Peerie moot, baby. Peerie grain, a little bit. Peerie wise, careful. I love the dialect and often have a problem thinking up the proper English word.

'Would you like a cup of tea while you're waiting?'

'Oh, bless you,' says my father, 'I am definitely in need of a cuppa and I'm sure Mona is too.'

Christine disappears into the kitchen but remains within ear shot. As the welcome tea is brought, Christine continues, 'It takes the crew a bit to off-load the cargo, and then some time to load her up, so just relax while all this is going on. Mind, Mona, and go to the loo before you board, there's no toilet on the *Good Shepherd*'.

'What! No loo, Christine? But it's a three-hour journey,' I reply, sheepishly.

'Well, that's the way it is,' Christine is laughing. 'No fancy ferry for you, my lass. You'll either have to sit up on deck with the crew, or if you're feeling seasick there's always a bunk down below, and a bucket for any emergencies.' I feel my mouth drop open. 'Before the early 1920s there was no regular boat to and from Fair Isle, as folk seldom needed to leave.'

'Yes, I remember well when Fair Isle got the *Good Shepherd ll*, the very one you'll be going on, Mona; that was in 1937,' says dad. 'She's a mail boat and cargo vessel about 47 feet long, if I remember right, built on the lines of a fishing boat, and has never pretended to be a passenger ferry. I'm looking forward to seeing her. This is quite a day for me.'

'Let's go for a walk, Dad, and get a bit of fresh air.'

It's a beautiful, late summer's day. Shetland is at her best. Gulls are screaming over our heads, salt is in the air, a seal is bobbing far out to sea and, as we turn the corner there it is, a full rainbow with each of the seven stripes distinct and vivid. We both stand in awe.

'Rainbows are aye a good omen, lass. I think the good Lord has put that there especially for you.'

'I'm still not convinced, Dad.' My throat aches with unshed tears. I don't want to let him down by weeping. 'But I'm going to give it all I've got'.

'You were always the bairn who was up for an adventure. Well, here it is. You're going to the most remote inhabited isle of the British Isles. Crossing one of the most dangerous sea crossings, 25 sea miles it is. What could be more exciting than that? Come to think of it, I wish I was coming too.'

'Oh, how I wish you were,' I say, betraying more of my nervousness than I want to. 'But look. That must be the *Good Shepherd*!' Dad and I watch as she slides up to her mooring at the Grutness pier. In no time we see men in yellow oilskins offload cargo. Pulling dad's hand, I venture nearer to have a good look. The cargo hold is open and from another hold steps lead to what I take to be the crew's quarters.

A slightly-built man with hand already outstretched approaches. 'Are you passengers? I'm Jerry, skipper of the *Good Shepherd.*'

My father shakes the skipper's hand vigorously. 'I'm Charlie Smith. Meet my daughter Mona, she's your new island nurse. One of these days I'll be coming for a visit. Meantime, I hope you'll look after her.' Dad is smiling but I detect a degree of fatherly concern in his voice.

'We certainly will. She'll look after us and we'll look after her. Come, let me introduce you to the crew. These two are brothers, Alec and Georgie, and this is Jimmy, and here's Tommy.'

Four pairs of eyes look me up and down. I'm sure they're thinking, 'She's a bit young for the job'. Then, 'Welcome,' rings out in unison and broad smiles shine out from sun-browned faces while strong, calloused hands shake my peerie, soft one.

'Not long now, Nurse, and we'll be off,' Jerry pats my shoulder. 'You're the only passenger today. It's a bonnie day but of course Da Roost has to be crossed. I hope you're not seasick as Da Roost is always choppy. When you're ready, come aboard and take a seat on the bench.'

"Da Roost" is the current that we cross on the passage to Aberdeen. The ferry would buck and sway a little as it negotiated the current. But it is, dad explains to me, a little more hazardous travelling to Fair Isle. There, it's an unforgiving tidal race that forms the gap between Grutness and Fair Isle. The two tidal streams meet, causing a great churning of the water. It's this upheaval that makes many a person sick, but also provides the abundance of fish that in turn attract the dolphins and whales.

I give my dear dad a hug, wave to Christine, who is standing in the door waving back at me furiously, and I board the *Good Shepherd* without a backward glance.

CHAPTER 2

It's starting to drizzle now and I can tell from the dark clouds that have scudded up from the south that rain is on the way. The sea, though, is relatively calm and I decide to sit quietly on the bench on the deck of the *Good Shepherd* to watch the harbour disappear behind us.

Now that we are round the point of mainland Shetland and heading due south, I turn and look back. The scene is one of the Shetland history lessons I remember from my school days that literally has come to life before my very eyes. My favourite teacher, Mr Graham, had the knack of making all the lessons he taught exciting and often romantic. I hear his voice in my head:

Long ago, when the world was thought to be flat, a Greek explorer named Pytheas set out to find the edge of the world. He sailed on and on, ever north, until he found himself in a great expanse of empty, cheerless water. Just when he began to think that no more land existed, he noticed a break on the horizon, a great mass like a jagged tooth rose out of the ocean ...

By this time you could have heard a pin drop, as the whole class held a collective breath. Mr Graham certainly had a way of telling a story. He would pause, and then scan the class, adding to the drama:

This encouraged Pytheas to sail on.

Thank goodness for that, I remember thinking.

The sight of foam from giant waves hurling themselves against bastions guarding the unknown, met his eyes. Here again was land ...

Oh, yes, Mr Graham, now these points and promontories and foam are meeting my eyes thousands of years later. I spy Fitful Head, near the edge of a line of broken cliffs. Then Sumburgh Head, a 100-metre-high rocky cliff capped by the Sumburgh Lighthouse.

No lighthouse in your day, Mr Pytheas. Mr Graham was at great pains to tell us that you ordered your crew to turn around lest they sail into the abyss. This, you said, must be the edge of the world, and you named it Ultima Thule.

But you didn't have the last say, Pytheas.

Mr Graham went on: *Much later, the Vikings observed that the shape of the archipelago of islands looked like the hilt of a sword, and named it Hjaltland. Finally, the Scots took over and renamed it Shetland ... common old Shetland.*

I remember thinking ... spoilsports!

Thousands of sea birds swoop and dive off Sumburgh Head. I'm so taken up with the sight of Shetland disappearing that I've hardly noticed that the *Good Shepherd* has started to rear and dip in the most alarming way. The sea is no longer placid. It consists now of a series of enormous swells. Da Roost has struck with a vengeance and I realise I must lie down at once.

I meet Georgie coming out of the wheelhouse. 'I'll tak you doon below and maybe you'll settle and have a sleep. Seasickness is not fine at all. Not dat I ken onything aboot it, but I've seen plenty o it. Da Roost is a beggar, but we have to git ower her.'

Georgie helps me into a bottom bunk, places a pail nearby and a tin into my shaky hands. 'No very sophisticated but it should do da job. I have to git back to da wheelhoose, but I'll send een o da men doon to see du's aaricht.'

My head is pounding. I fumble for the vomit basin, or should I say the old National Dried Milk tin. The worn blanket, which Georgie has tenderly covered me with, offers little. The stink – a mixture of old vomit, fumes from the engine and diesel oil – is enough to make anyone sick, regardless of the state of the ocean. I hear the crew above chatting and laughing amongst themselves. Hardy islanders they certainly are and, from what I saw of them on the Grutness pier, they seem a caring lot.

A moan escapes my mouth. My empty stomach has no more to offer. My body heaves in sync with the boat's motion. Then Alec appears. 'Now, dunna you worry, I'll keep my eye on you,' he says, as he firmly holds my head and holds the tin. I half open my eyes to thank him. Even in my pathetic state I can make out his knowing sea-blue eyes holding mine.

After what seems like ages, the motion beneath us calms as the boat chugs out of da infamous Roost and makes for home. Dehydration and exhaustion lull me into a troubled sleep.

I am wakened by the clanging of chains and a cacophony of shouting and laughter. I tentatively swing my feet to the floor. My legs nearly give way but Alec is once again by my side.

I see Georgie's beaming face at the top of the stairs. 'We're nearly dere, Nurse, I'm vexed you wir sae seek, but it's just the wye o it.' His arm reaches down to give me a hand up, as Alec leads me to the top deck.

I close my eyes and I gulp in great lungfuls of pure fresh air. Georgie hands me a bottle of water, I drink, and I'm amazed that nothing more down there wants to come up. I am refreshed. Standing on my own two feet the wind lifts my hair, and the afternoon sun warms my face. I open my eyes to a scene so awe-inspiring it lies permanently imprinted in my mind.

Great towering cliffs reach to the heavens and a clear blue neverending sea stretches to the far horizon. The sheer natural beauty, despite the foul taste in my mouth, causes me to gasp. Arctic terns call a welcome and the multi-coloured beaks of the puffins shyly peep out from their burrows high in the cliffs. The white sand of North Haven lies ahead of me. It's a picture-postcard scene for sure, but that doesn't stop the butterflies from fluttering in the pit of my tummy. I try hard to stifle my trepidation as Alec approaches, offering his help with my luggage.

Alec walks ahead of me down the narrow gangway carrying my heavy suitcase. The air is full of the cries and laughter of a number of children playing on the shore. He sets down the case and turns to me. 'It's a bit of a climb up top, Nurse, then my auld pick-up can take us to your house, but you'll have to wait a bit. I need to go back and give the men a hand with tying up and off-loading.'

'There's a lot of folk about, Alec. What are they here for? Certainly not to meet passengers, and I'm sure not to meet me.'

'Oh no, they would never be so forward. They're here to pick up their orders from the mainland, and just for a jaunt to see what's going on.'

'Yun most be da new nurse,' a young lad shouts to his friend. It never fails to amaze me that in Shetland's population of 18,000 souls, there are so many different versions of the Shetland dialect.

I give the children a big wave and shout back, 'Yes, you're right, dat's me. I'm Mona, your nurse.'

It's good to be out in the fresh air and to stretch my legs on the climb up from the harbour to the rough track on which Alec's pick-up stands. The threatened storm hasn't reached Fair Isle, and the sun is warm as I lean against the old pick-up that has certainly seen better days. I'm grateful for his offer of a lift as I don't fancy a walk. My legs are still a bit shaky.

I look back at the forbidding cliffs around North Haven and I think again about my dad, who constantly assured me that I could pull this off, but yet again I doubt myself and wonder if I'm up to the task. A whole year on this tiny island? Won't I go mad with loneliness? Will I be able to cope with the medical emergencies that will doubtlessly challenge me? Will the islanders accept me? I take a deep breath and consciously dismiss these negative thoughts from my mind.

CHAPTER 3

Alec trudges up from the jetty lugging my suitcase. He dumps it in the back of the pick-up and then opens the passenger door for me. 'The Rayburn is on and there's plenty of hot water.' Alec, with the open, friendly face, blond hair and blue eyes that suggest our Viking ancestry.

'Are you a Fair Isle man?' I ask.

'Oh yes, I am. Margaret, my wife, is from Lerwick, and she has settled down to the ways of the isle, but not everyone does, so I am hoping you will. We have two peerie boys, Michael and Kenneth. You'll be visiting us soon, I hope?'

'I look forward to meeting the Fair Isle folk and your family too.'

Five minutes on our way, I see on my left a distinctive rock rising out of the sea. I recognise this from photographs as Fair Isle's most distinctive feature.

'Alec,' I remark, with excitement in my voice, 'is that the Sheep Rock?'

'Yes, it is. I'll stop da car and I'll join dee for a good look. The folk fae sooth tell us it's "iconic", I'm no too sure about dat, but what I can tell dee is it's hard work getting the sheep up and doon da cliff.'

Alec goes on to tell me more. The Sheep Rock is 132 metres high and, from where we are standing, he points out steeply sloping grass on top of a rocky outcrop. It looks like a grass ski slope. I am amazed that there are sheep on top of this strange looking rock.

'Alec!' I exclaim, 'why on earth would you put sheep on such a dangerous place?'

'Well, Fair Isle needs every precious blade of grass to feed the sheep, and up on tap there's four hectares that mustn't go to waste.'

'And how do you get them up there, let alone down? Surely you risk life and limb?'

I can tell Alec is highly amused at my questions. He gives a jolly laugh before answering. 'We've been doing this for centuries. Mind you, if we do fall, dat will become dy problem. I'm joking wi dee, it's never happened yet. We row out and three men climb the face and secure the ropes. On the last bit o da climb there's a chain, that wir forebears lang fae syne rigged up, to give a bit more safety. Da ropes are let doon and the men at the bottom tie the sheep, one by one, and up they go.'

I'm taking a peerie start to process this information. Well, dad did say life here would be a challenge. We both fall silent until we reach my cottage and my bags are carried in and a good night's sleep is on the cards. But first I need to know how I will be contacted if needed.

'Not to worry, Nurse, they know where to find you if they need you.' That charming lilt again, with no barrage of questions asked, and I have no energy left to ask the hundred and one I need answered.

I have no preconceived ideas about my new home; what I see is what I get. I prowl around, and it suddenly strikes me that I never enquired about my living arrangements. I know the house was purpose-built by the local authority, as are all the district nurses' houses throughout Shetland – somewhat boring, somewhat utility. I am surprised, though, by a garden and yard area, two double bedrooms, a bathroom, a nice big kitchen and a sitting room with a view that I am sure has been there since time began, with no man-made intrusion, just the sea and the cliffs. The clear blue sky with a few white fluffy clouds far above holds me entranced. Tired as I am, I make a mental note to explore this bonnie isle.

The house is spacious and I'm thinking that, in the past, there must have been nurses with large families living here. I'll bounce around like a marble in a pinball machine. At least I can have friends and family to visit. That's if they can tackle the crossing.

I see a door off the kitchen with a bold "CLINIC" written in capital letters, and a strange looking phone with a handle on a shelf beside the door. By this time I'm too tired to think. For the next year, 70 human beings will depend on me to keep them healthy and care for them when they are ill.

'Sufficient unto the day is the evil thereof,' is my last thought as I climb into a big comfortable bed and fall into a deep, dreamless sleep.

CHAPTER 4

I awake to the sun streaming into my bedroom. August, of course, is one of Shetland's sunniest months and I had forgotten to pull the curtains. For at least five seconds I have no idea where I am, then reality strikes and I jump out of bed.

During the summer months in Shetland, if the sky is clear it never gets really dark. At midsummer the sun will set at around 10.30pm and will rise again around 3.30am. The five hours in between are a time of prolonged dusk, known in Shetland as the simmer dim: nineteen hours of sunshine. If the sky remains clear, there is enough light to read outside the entire night. By contrast, at midwinter there are fewer than six hours of daylight.

I scramble for my watch. Quarter past four. Is this morning or afternoon, I think for a second? Then smile at my confusion. Oh well, since I'm already wide awake I decide to have a look around the kitchen. Good: tea and coffee, a jug of milk, bread and butter, eggs, too. I open the Rayburn door, the embers still look promising so I shovel in some coal, give it a stir and in no time at all the kettle is singing. I realise I'm hungry and remember that I was too tired to eat last night.

My tummy has settled at last so, after a king-sized breakfast, I take a mug with a lovely picture of a puffin on the outside and steaming coffee on the inside, sit on the kitchen steps and take in my surroundings. The first thing I see is a Shetland ewe tethered to a stake on my front lawn. 'Now who are you, bonnie lady, and where did you come from? I'm thrilled to have you for company.' I'm sure if she could smile she would give me a huge one.

Right. I give myself a shake, it's time to get to grips with my new life.

CHAPTER 5

The Zetland County Council health department is leaving nothing to chance. This reassuring thought sustains me as I rummage around the clinic room. Well-stocked cupboards contain the latest medicines, syringes of all sizes, bandages and dressings. An oxygen cylinder, fracture boards, sutures that could fix a pony let alone a human, and a first response bag for an emergency.

I'm intrigued with the paraffin fridge, and as I open the door and see the vaccines inside I suddenly remember that there is no electricity on the isle.

All the working tools are in order but, as I close the cupboards, suddenly a vision of childbirth comes to mind. Will I cope with all that is expected? I know I have to get the pregnant ladies off the isle to the maternity section of the Gilbert Bain Hospital in Lerwick at 36 weeks. But, what if? Suddenly I find myself surrounded by 'what ifs'. Premature labour? Pregnancy bleeding? The *Good Shepherd* can't go because of the storm? An accident on the treacherous cliffs causing haemorrhage and broken bones?

I take a deep breath and get down on my knees. I am a Christian girl, but life has come between me and my faith. I haven't been on my knees in ages. Suddenly I feel foolish. My pride battles with my humility. Thank God humility wins.

'Dear Lord Jesus, I am here alone. The nearest medical help is far away, a good four hours if the weather is kind. You know that already, Lord, why do I think you need me to tell you? I'm depending on you. Guide my thoughts, my hands and my tongue so that I never say or do anything that can hurt another. I am depending totally upon you and if there is any glory attached to this, then it is all to you. I pray, in your name, Amen.'

I get to my feet. It's now 7.00am and I decide to take a good look at the funny phone I noticed last night. I have never seen a phone with a handle before and have no idea of how this strange implement is supposed to work. I lift the receiver and hear a dialling tone. Good! That's promising. I replace the receiver. I'll have to get to grips with this thing as it's a lifeline between me and Dr Mainland. His GP practice is at Levenwick, not far from Grutness, and he is the doctor responsible for Fair Isle. I must talk to him and introduce myself.

This thought has no sooner passed through my brain than I hear a knock at my door. A small neat woman with a beaming smile is standing there. What I immediately notice is her eyes. The more she smiles, the more they disappear into her kind happy face.

'I'm Annie, your next door neighbour. You must be Nurse Smith.'

'I am,' I say. We shake hands. She has a firm grip. 'Oh, do come in, Annie. I'll make you a cup of tea, or maybe coffee?

'I'm a real tea-jenny, so tea will be great.' Annie plonks herself down at the kitchen table and as I busy myself with the tea making, Annie tells me that Stewart, her husband, helps her run the post office, and her son, also Stewart, is in charge of the telephone exchange. She reassures me that husband Stewart will make sure my house is well maintained and that they both filled my cupboards, and will help me settle in.

'Thank you very much, Annie, I'm blyde to meet you. I have many questions. What is it with this funny phone?'

'That's what has sent me in. I could hear you had lifted the receiver, and then nothing. So I thought it best to come and let you know how it works. We're on a party-line during the day. Just lift the receiver and turn the handle and I'll make contact for you. Incoming calls – one ring it's for the post office, and three rings it's for you. From seven o'clock in the evening 'til nine in the morning you'll be able to dial straight through.'

My goodness me, I'm thinking, I'll have to process this information. At least in an emergency I'll be able to make contact with the outside world, day and night. Annie continues. 'There are not many phones on the isle, but we do have a public phone box outside the post office.'

Poor Annie is at the receiving end of my many questions; she is a gracious woman, in her forties I'm thinking, and she answers each one fully and faithfully.

'That's your safe there, Nurse.'

'Oh, Annie, "Nurse"? I know I will have to be known as "Nurse", and it won't be everybody I'll invite to call me Mona, but please, if you will, I would like that.'

'Of course, thank you, Mona.'

Annie gives me a quick and efficient tour of my house, including the safe and the medical records drawer and so forth. She explains that Dr Mainland visits the isle from time to time. And then she says something that sends a shiver up my spine. 'If he learns to trust you, he'll come less and less.'

I don't know what to think as Annie continues. 'I'm not sure if your superiors told you what to expect here, so if I start to tell you something that you already know, stop me. You have no car, of course, but then the isle is only three miles long and one and a half wide, so that shouldn't be a problem with your young legs. In an emergency, or if you need transport urgently, call on Stewart and he'll look after you.'

Annie is in no hurry and she kindly fills me in on my immediate outdoor environment. She tells me that most of the houses and crofts are in this area on the south side, the arable side of the isle. The north side, apparently, is not much use for anything but sheep.

The bird observatory, near North Haven, is run by Roy Dennis. Three families live in the North Lighthouse. 'It's a long walk,' she warns me, 'but if you need to go in a hurry, or during the night, you can call on Stewart.'

'Thanks again, Annie, I'm beginning to get the picture. You and Stewart must be a godsend for the nurses coming in here. Miss Williamson, my superior in Lerwick, is a family friend and she was so taken up with persuading me to come to Fair Isle that she didn't give me a lot of information. What she did do, was persuade my dad to persuade me.' Annie bursts out laughing. 'And here I am, Annie. I hope I'm up for this. She did say I was to get on with things, find my own way, and if I needed to ask questions I should phone her, not that she filled me in about the handle.' Now we're both laughing.

Annie goes on to reassure me that the isle folk will give me every encouragement and support. 'By the way, the shop is next door on the other side of this house. Stewart Wilson – yes, before you ask, another Stewart – him and his wife Sheila, she's from Orkney by the way, oh yes, and pregnant – I'm not gossiping now, it's common knowledge – she'll be a customer for you. Well, Sheila and Stewart run the well-stocked shop, so you shouldn't be deprived of the finer things of life.'

CHAPTER 6

I begin to worry that I'm taking up too much of Annie's time. After all, she must be a busy woman running the post office. I voice my concern and am reassured that she is enjoying our chat. She suggests another cup of tea. While I'm busy, she goes back home for the tray of bannocks she baked earlier. In no time, Annie and I are at my kitchen table enjoying homemade bannocks slathered with home-kirned butter.

'That's good news, Annie, about the shop, but a baby on the way, that's right up my street. I love midwifery. I have to admit I feel a bit cheated that I have to hand over the mums to the hospital in Lerwick. Not that I disagree with the policy. A home birth in Fair Isle would be far too risky.'

Annie goes on to tell me about times when there was no nurse on the isle and the mothers and aunts delivered the babies. 'I mind once, I was only a bairn then,' – Annie's face tautens with the memory – 'there was a trained nurse and midwife here, but when the mother went into labour there were big problems. Obstructed labour, I think it was. The *Good Shepherd* went to fetch the doctor from Levenwick.

I mind the folk saying the doctor attempted a caesarean, but too late. The mam and baby both died. Sandy never got over the tragedy. You'll meet him.'

I shiver. 'That's a terrible story, Annie. I am so blyde things have moved on. Are there any more pregnancies for me to care for?'

'We have to be very careful here, Mona, about hearsay and gossip. You'll find out once you read the medical records and notes. Sheila is well on, so it's common knowledge about her baby, but as for the rest, I can't say.

'Ah, thanks, Annie, point taken. Confidentiality is my middle name.'

Annie and I go on chatting and she tells me a bit about herself. Munching on her bannocks, I feel completely comfortable in her company. She tells me she and her husband Stewart have three bairns. Anne, the eldest, is a teacher in Shetland, her youngest is at the Anderson Institute – the high school in Lerwick. Only her middle boy, Stewart, remains with them on the island, running the telephone exchange. 'He's a dyed-in-the-wool Fair Isle boy,' she says. We giggle at the pun because, of course, I already know that Fair Isle is known as much for its wool and stranded knitting style, as it is for its wildlife and rugged scenery.

Annie goes on to tell me that young Stewart is about my age and she hopes we will become friends. She misses her son, Neil, one of the seven Fair Isle children who live in the school hostel in Lerwick. This hostel caters for children from outlying areas in Shetland. 'We do enjoy great celebrations when the bairns come home for the school holidays. They'll be home for Christmas. It's hard for the young ones, leaving the isle at only 12.'

I am about to give Annie an answer when there's a light knock on the kitchen door and a tall, good-looking man enters, with a broad smile. 'Thought it best if I came in and introduced myself. I'm Stewart, Annie's better half.'

I take his strong hand. 'Annie's been filling me in on the ways of Fair Isle. But I can hear by your accent that you're not a Fair Isle man.'

'No, you're right, I'm from Unst. That's the most northerly isle in Shetland ... ' I am already nodding because everyone from our part of the world knows Unst, because of its traditional gossamer lace knitwear. 'And before you ask, I came here as a young lighthouse keeper, met my lovely Annie and the rest is history.'

I like Stewart's candid manner, and a man who is not timid about giving his wife a compliment is my kind of man.

'Oh, by the way, what's with the ewe staked on my lawn? She's a Shetland breed, I see.'

'This peerie ewe lost her mother, so we took her in. I tether her on your lawn, and keep moving her so she has fine, fresh green grass to eat. You do have a lawn mower in the shed, but this arrangement makes far more sense. If it's okay with you, Caddy can earn her keep by us giving you a jug of milk every day.'

I tell Stewart I'm happy with this arrangement as I don't know one end of a lawn mower from the other, and that I'm in love with Caddy already. 'I trust she's not for my Sunday roast?' Both Annie and Stewart give a smile but no answer.

Then Annie says, 'Stewart and I will keep an eye out for you. It's still bonnie weather, maybe a walk will clear the cobwebs. That's Malcolm's Head you can see from the window. A walk up to the top, then along to the South Lighthouse, and back along the road will do you the world of good. We'll have to get going, anyway. If you do decide on the walk, leave the key with us, and mind, come along for your tea tonight.'

CHAPTER 7

I don a pair of walking boots, jeans and a light jersey and I'm off. I love walking, and striding out in fresh, unpolluted air is a true blessing after my previous post in the smog of Glasgow. The grass is soft under my feet. Rabbits scuttle as I approach. Buttercups, daisies and violets remind me of childhood days, when we picked bunches of these beauties from beside the road on our way home from school.

I climb over a couple of stiles and, as I look up into a clear blue sky, I wonder how long this fine weather will last, and decide to enjoy every minute of it while it's on offer. I'm only too aware how it can change. A feeling of happiness overtakes me as I realise how blessed I am to be part of nature's story and, because no one is near to hear me, I sing one of my favourite Beatles songs, *Please, Please, Me* at the top of my voice.

It's a challenging climb and I'm out of breath by the time I reach the top of Malcolm's Head, due, I dare say, to the singing as much as the climbing. I have no idea who Malcolm is, or was. I make a mental note to ask Annie. This thought is suddenly replaced by the breathtaking vista that meets my eyes. Out west, there's nothing between me and

America. Below are two sheer cliffs, with sea birds ducking and diving and disappearing into what, I'm guessing, are secret ledges in the cliff face, where they will nest and nurture their young.

I am glad to see that the thousands of puffins are still with us, birds that faithfully return to the same mate, and the same burrow, every summer to lay their eggs and start a new generation of Tammie Norries, as they are called in Shetland. They will wait until their chicks are fledged before leaving. I love the Tammie Norries. Shy birds they are, but I do spy two, maybe husband and wife? I smile at my imaginings. Since childhood, they have never failed to entertain me with their clown-like masks and strange waddling gait. Next time, I promise myself, I will bring my camera.

Meanwhile, I'm soaking up the spectacle of the two cliffs separated by an inlet, sheltering a spectacular sea stack rising vertically out of the ocean. I see more sea stacks further out, but this one is fascinating. It's the spitting image of a side-on view of Queen Victoria, complete with crown.

On my way once more, towards the South Lighthouse. A wooden shed comes into view and, as I approach, a young man emerges. It's Tommy Stout, whom I recognise as one of the crew of the *Good Shepherd.*

'Hello, Nurse, I see you're out and about on this bonnie day. How's it going with you? Settling in, I hope.'

'I'm trying my best to take everything in, but that's going to take some time. My head and my eyes are so full of the scenes and wonders of your bonnie isle. Oh, there's the South Lighthouse, I'm off down for a look, and then it's back up the road to my house.'

'I'm just on my wye down, too. If you don't mind, I'll join you.'

'Oh, yes, it's good to have a bit of company. Tell me, what's this shed doing here, spoiling the landscape?' I say this with tongue in cheek and a smile, as I don't want to offend. This old shed might be of importance to the isle, and to Tommy himself.

Tommy has a strong-featured face, the kind of face you trust instantly. He has a booming voice and a hearty laugh that puts me right at ease. Sure enough, the shed had, and still has, a vital role to play, as Tommy explains.

'This old shed, as you call her, was manned day and night during the First World War. Enemy ships, or any ship in distress, were reported to my grand-uncle Jaarm, whose duty it was to inform the Admiralty by Morse code.'

'Morse code, gosh, that sounds so old-fashioned.'

'Well, the same practice applied during the last war, but by then Uncle Jaarm made contact by phone.'

I'm duly impressed. I peep through the door and see a phone, complete with handle, looking incongruous in the corner. I also note a paraffin heater and a big pair of binoculars in amongst a clutter of other paraphernalia.

Tommy points to a white double-storey house far to the south. 'That's Ootra, as we call it, or Melville House, the posh name,' another laugh rings out. 'Uncle Jaarm is long dead but his two daughters, Helen and Lottie, still live there. You'll be visiting them.'

'I do look forward to getting to know them. They must be quite old?'

'They are getting on a bit, but don't ever suggest that to them. They manage fine and the whole community looks out for them.'

Tommy lifts a hand to shade his eyes and scans the horizon. 'We're still on call here if the weather turns bad. No need today, so I'm taking this time to make sure everything's in order.'

'But Tommy, do you do on-call duty? You're part of the *Good Shepherd* crew, so how does that work?'

Tommy gives me a quizzical look. 'It's a peerie place, so we all take turns at whatever needs doing. I'm also a part-time lighthouse keeper, and can take over when a keeper is ill or goes on holiday. I also help mum and dad run our croft – that's Busta, ower dere,' Tommy points to a house on the far east of the isle.

South Lighthouse comes to view, a pristine building with foghorns and an impressive tower.

'Gosh, Tommy!' I exclaim. 'What a beautiful sight. I've never been this close to a lighthouse.'

Tommy goes on to tell me the light has guided ships and mariners since 1892, and that Fair Isle is blessed to have two of them, the other being on the north point of the isle. 'Much need, as you can imagine. Before the days of lighthouses there were many shipwrecks. There's accommodation in there for three keepers and their families. That's a good thing as it boosts the population and the bairns keep the school going.'

'Oh, yes, the school, I must find out about that.'

Tommy tells me there are eight bairns in the school and that they are now back at their classes after the long summer holidays. He continues to point out various landmarks. 'There's the cemetery, or kirk yard as we call it. The South Harbour, where the Royal Yacht *Britannia* anchored to let Queen Elizabeth and Prince Phillip disembark so that they could visit the isle. That wiz a few years fae syne, 1960 if I mind right. My mum will fill dee in aboot the visit.' Tommy is smiling at the memory.

The whitewashed crofts along the road back to my house look like dolls' houses from where I'm standing. They appear so comfortable and, nestled where they are, with their vegetable yards blossoming and their dry stone dykes, they are a joy to behold.

As we near the lighthouse, Tommy goes on to tell me that it was a ready target for enemy planes during the Second World War. The accommodation was hit in 1942, killing a keeper's wife and daughter.

'That's so sad to hear, Tommy. Thank you for your company and your stories about da isle.'

'Time I was on my way. I need to get back to my crofting duties.' With an engaging smile and a wave, Tommy strides off, leaving me to continue my hike.

CHAPTER 8

Everyone I've met so far has been so kind and accommodating. I begin to believe that perhaps I really will settle in here. Yes, my duties already seem less daunting and I really think I might manage very well.

I reach the road and am about to turn and make for home when a young woman runs towards me from the lighthouse. 'Are you the new nurse?' she asks, with a worried expression on her face.

'Yes, I am, can I help you?'

'I'm so glad you're here, I was about to phone your house. You see, my wee Millie is ill. She's very hot and doesn't want to eat or drink. She's miserable, and that's not like her, she's usually a happy wee lass.'

'I'll come in and see her straight away, Mrs ...?'

'I'm Mrs McPherson. My husband, Jack, is one of the keepers. Yes, please do come in, I can't tell you how glad I am you're here.'

The approach to the lighthouse is well maintained and the house clean and well kept. Millie's bedroom is bright and airy with lots of pictures and soft toys on display.

I make the visit as brief as possible as I need to go back home and fetch my medical bag. I feel Millie's forehead and try hard to reassure this wee girl and her mum. 'I can feel you're very hot, Millie. I'm Nurse Smith and I'll come straight back and give you medicine to make you better.'

Millie opens her eyes and gives me a smile and a nod, and immediately I am carried back to my own childhood. I was around Millie's age when I became suddenly ill at home in South Whiteness ...

Snowflakes were still falling outside the kitchen window, but sporadically now, almost apologetically. A bit late, Mr Snowman, I thought, to feel sorry for the blizzard that brought traffic to a standstill for much of the day and the night that followed.

It was left to the crew of the stalwart little fishing boat Budding Rose *to bring the doctor. Three hours it took, and from the relieved faces looking down at me I knew that his arrival was none too soon.*

The astringent smell of him made me open my painful eyes. There he was, smiling and bending over my crib. I tried to smile back, but everything hurt. I'd seen Dr Durham (or Dr Dubbin, as I called him) many times during my short life, since I suffered from a 'bad chest'. His appearance, immaculate as ever, with a starched collar, familiar cravat and soft leather gloves, reassured me that all would be well.

'Now, how's my peerie lass?' Dr Durham was a Shetlander, born and bred. The stethoscope was cold on my burning chest. 'I'm afraid it's pneumonia, Mrs Smith.' My mum's face showed concern, but one pat on her shoulder was all it took for her smile to come back.

The needle slid into my flesh with a sharp sting. I yelled my protest, but my mum's kiss on my four-year-old head was all the comfort I needed.

Snuggling into my blanket, I rolled over as the hiss of the kettle on the hob, the smell of the peat fire, the tick-tock of the American clock above my head, all lulled me to sleep ...

I tell Mrs McPherson not to give Millie any medicine and advise her to sponge her down with tepid water. I reassure her that I'll be back in a jiffy, then I hurry back to the house and freshen up, exchange my hiking clothes for a nurse's uniform and check my medical bag. On the way out, I pass Stewart and let him know where I'm off to and why. The wind is strengthening and I have to push against it as I walk, from time to time breaking into a half-run.

Back in Millie's bedroom, I take her temperature. The thermometer reads 99.5F and her tonsils are so large she can hardly speak. Wee trooper that she is, she tells me she's nearly four, and tries her best to cooperate as I prise her mouth open with the tongue depressor.

'Now, Millie, this is called a stethoscope. I need to listen to your chest, if you don't mind. It will probably feel cold.'

Millie tries to smile, bless her, and I'm glad to hear there's no sign of a chest infection. Her neck glands are up, but her tummy is soft and there's no sign of a rash. The diagnosis seems clear to me, but first I'll have to consult with Dr Mainland.

As I make my way home, it's a relief to have the wind at my back, helping me on my way. I lift the receiver, tentatively turn the handle and am relieved to hear Annie. 'Please put me through to Dr Mainland, Annie.' Gosh this really works.

I don't have to wait long to hear his deep voice on the other side. 'Hello Doctor, this is Nurse Smith here from Fair Isle.'

'Hello there, Nurse Smith, I'm so pleased that you've called me as I had every intention of phoning you today. I do hope you are settling in? You're a Shetlander, I believe, so that will help you understand the dialect and the ways of Fair Isle.'

'Yes, thank you, Doctor, so far so good.' I go on to discuss Millie's condition. Dr Mainland seems approachable, and listens intently as I reel off Millie's signs and symptoms.

'I also think it's tonsillitis. We'll go ahead with the pain relievers and the antibiotics. If you're worried, or she deteriorates, come back to me. Otherwise, give me a call tomorrow.'

I replace the receiver and, out of the blue it hits me. Or should I say the tension that has been building up over the past week bubbles up in my throat. I realise in a split second that I have been burying my worries deep within me. Not healthy, I tell myself and, at last, I give myself permission to have a good cry. Sitting down at the clinic table, I put my head in my hands and bawl my eyes out. All the pent-up tension comes pouring out of me.

Eventually, I dry my eyes and gaze out of the clinic window. Who in the world would not be enchanted by that view? I take a few minutes to enjoy what many folk in the inner cities of Britain and beyond would give their eye teeth for. Life comes into perspective. I feel my confidence return and I say a prayer of thanksgiving. Smiling through my tears, I square my shoulders and am on my way back to Millie, with a spring in my step.

I'm met by an anxious Mrs McPherson. 'You've had a busy morning, Nurse, and you must be hungry. I've got soup and fresh bread on the go, you're most welcome to join me. Jack is at the lighthouse. I'm so glad you're here to help Millie, and I can be doing with a bit of company.'

The soup and homemade bread are delicious and I can see Mrs McPherson is pleased when I ask for the recipe. The afternoon flows easily after that. It's good to have a chat and it gives me time to observe Millie, who is happy to sip water. As the medicine takes effect, she brightens and I explain to her about the antibiotic medication. She nods her head and in no time she's fast asleep.

I have a sixth sense that Mrs McPherson has something more on her mind. Several times she takes a deep breath, and then lets it out again. At first, I think she's concerned about Millie, but as she continues to bite her lip and fidget with her fingers, I'm positive that something else is worrying her. I bide my time and keep silent. Eventually, she rises and puts on the kettle. Standing at the counter, she turns and faces me.

'Nurse, I have something to tell you. I'm pregnant. Can't say I'm over the moon about it ...' Her voice breaks. 'It's an extra mouth to feed and, although Jack is well-compensated as a lighthouse keeper, life just seems to be one continuous wheel of cooking and cleaning. Jack is thrilled with another baby on the way. Sorry, Nurse, I didn't mean to cry.'

Remembering my own recent bout of tears, a wave of sympathy comes over me. I put my arms around this sobbing woman and reassure her that I have all the time in the world.

She goes on to tell me what her real concern is. She thinks she had a 'bit' of postnatal depression after Millie was born. At the time she didn't tell the nurse, who was a much older woman, as she didn't want to burden her. 'In fact,' she goes on between the sobs, 'I didn't want to burden anyone. I know Jack was worried about me, but we just got on with it, and eventually I came right. Now I'm worried it might start up again after this baby's born.'

I let Margaret – by now we're on first-name terms – cry her worries out. During the next couple of hours I learn that she is eight weeks pregnant. I am able to reassure her that I will look after her during her pregnancy and will still be on the isle when she has her baby.

I'm guessing, but I'm sure what Margaret is in need of is a bit of mothering. I'm much younger than she is, but that doesn't matter. I find a nice fat cushion, then encourage her to sit in the big upholstered armchair. I tuck the cushion behind her back and lift her feet up onto a low stool.

'You're so kind, Nurse. I'm feeling heaps better already.' Her pretty face lights up as she smiles.

'I'm glad you told me about your depression after Millie was born.' I go on to reassure her that I trained as a midwife in a big teaching hospital in London and studied this condition. 'I'll tell Dr Mainland, and I'm sure we'll work out a plan for you. I'll be checking on Millie daily, and I'll give you an antenatal check tomorrow when I'm here.' I'm relieved to see a glimmer of a smile when I say, 'Keep me a specimen of your urine, you know the score.'

We have another cup of tea while I listen to Margaret tell me about her life, and about being a lighthouse keeper's wife. Her family live on the Scottish mainland and she often gets homesick. By the time I leave, I'm satisfied that both Millie and mum Margaret are doing okay.

'Thank you, Nurse.' The smile is widening. 'It's a big relief to get this off my chest. I look forward to your visit tomorrow.'

Lying back in a hot bubble bath, I reflect on my first day as district nurse in Fair Isle. It's been quite a day. Whoever it was who warned me that I would find it boring to spend a year stuck on a treeless, windswept rock in the middle of the unpredictable water between the North Sea and the Atlantic Ocean didn't know what they were talking about

I feel myself drifting dreamily away, but am awoken by the rattle of rain against the window pane.

CHAPTER 9

I'm so relaxed, I'm about to drift off again, when I remember that I have an invitation to tea. I hop out of the bath, dry myself, throw on my jeans and a warm cardigan and make my way next door, through the pouring rain.

I look up as I enter and see the word 'Shirva' carved on a piece of driftwood above the door. It's a sign that will grow familiar to me over the months ahead, and I will learn that, in local dialect, it means a 'high, rocky place near water'.

I give a peerie knock and walk in to a cosy, homely livingroom-cum-kitchen.

'Come in, come in,' Annie greets me with her bright infectious smile. 'You had to go back to the lighthouse, Stewart tells me, so you've had a busy day of it.'

'My lips are sealed, Annie.' We both laugh. 'Yes, I have had a busy day, but a good day. It's so fine to come in and have my tea with you, thank you again for the unexpected invitation.'

Stewart welcomes me in. He announces that Annie has made one of her famous steak and kidney pies with rhubarb crumble to follow. He is wearing a Fair Isle jersey, which I remark on. 'The colours seem so natural, hardly dyed at all. But my mouth is watering already, Stewart. I'm starving.'

'So am I.' He suggests that we first have our tea and then Annie will give me the low-down on the maakin, which is how Shetland folk refer to their particular style of knitting.

And so the three of us comfortably continue our conversation in our native tongue while we demolish the delicious food. Eventually, we lean back, completely sated. 'Annie,' I say, 'dat wiz joost delicious, me belly is stentit, I'll need tae watch oot else I'll be as fat as a selkie afore I ken o' it.'

I'm only too happy to give a hand with the washing up. There's plenty of hot water on tap, and I take note of the two-ring Calor gas cooker, like the one I have next door. It's a handy addition to the solid fuel stove.

'There's the generator clicking in,' says Stewart, 'did you hear it last night?'

'I heard nothing. I went out like a light. But speaking of lights, before I fell asleep, I tried all the electric switches and nothing happened.'

'Sorry, Mona, we should have told you.' Stewart goes on to explain that Fair Isle depends on diesel generators for its basic electrical needs.

A wave of nausea threatens to overpower me as I remember the diesel oil smell on the *Good Shepherd*. I take a big deep breath and focus on what Stewart is telling me. 'Not much need now in summer for electric lights, so the generator will kick in at seven and go off at 11. Don't miss out if you need to do a spot of ironing. During winter, it's 3.30pm till 11.'

Annie is busy maakin, clicking away at lightning speed. Without looking at what she is doing, she joins the conversation. I watch her carefully as she pushes the holding wire firmly into her maakin belt.

'Fine belt you have there, Annie, but it looks well used, you must be a busy woman, and by the way, that jersey you're working on is truly a work of art.'

'Well, as you know, no Shetland woman worth her salt is without her maakin belt and neither does she maak in pieces and then sew them up to create a garment, like the south folk do. We maak it all in one. But you ken aa that. Do you maak?'

'Yes, I do. Mind you, we all learn at our mother's knee. Some are better at it than others, and I'm definitely in the "others" camp. Mam and my sisters are lovely Fair Isle knitters, but as for me, I haven't worn a belt or touched a wire in years. I've been south for the last eight years, learning to be a nurse. Looking at you, Annie, and this bonnie maakin, I'm vexed I didn't keep up. Maybe you could give me a few lessons.'

'That would be such a pleasure. Come du in onytime du his a minute to spare, and if I'm at my "sok", du can watch and learn.'

I laugh at sok, another word for knitting or maakin. 'Thanks, Annie, I'll take you up on it.'

And so, a couple of hours slip past as I admire the many beautiful garments Annie has produced. Stewart has been busy settling down the hens and the croft in general. When he joins us again, he brings a beautifully crafted spinning wheel. He tells me that he loves making spinning wheels as well as spinning the wool.

'I had no idea there would be such talent right on my doorstep. I can see I'm not going to be bored. You never know, I might become a crack hand at the Fair Isle maakin, and maybe become a spinner to boot.'

With that, the door bursts open and in comes a young man, whom I realise immediately must be Stewart junior. He turns out to be as genial as his parents and tells me it's good to have a young nurse on the isle and he hopes we will become friends. He knows the place like the back of his hand and suggests that it would be a great pleasure to show me around.

'You folks are far too kind. Now I'm being offered a free tour guide. I'll certainly take you up on it. Now, though, I really must be on my way, it's time for bed. I'm tired, so goodnight and again thank you for your care and hospitality.'

Wow, this has been quite a day. My thoughts whirl as rain lashes my bedroom window and mixed emotions tumble through my head.

There is enough of the Shetlander in me to know that the best way to approach, and get to know, the Shetland folk is to spend time with them. But this does take time and, although they are friendly and warm, they don't give their hearts away until you have proved you are sincere and genuine. They don't countenance banal small talk. I realise that I will have to visit each household in Fair Isle and take the time to listen and communicate on a deep level.

Instead of worrying about not getting to sleep, I reflect on my first working day. It's barely 24 hours since I arrived. Much has happened: a sick child, a pregnant woman, my conversation with Dr Mainland, not to mention my thoughts on postnatal depression. I fall asleep finally, thinking about young Stewart's offer to be my tour guide. Tammie Norries, Queen Victoria and Royal yachts fill my dreams.

CHAPTER 10

Three months have now passed and, strange as it may seem, even to my own mind, I've been busy, with little time to think about 'me'. It's now a lazy Sunday in November, cold and drab, with a few sleet showers.

This morning, along with every able-bodied islander, I dress in my Sunday best and set off to da kirk. Fair Isle has no fewer than two churches, offering two services every Sunday. Two churches, I'm thinking, for seventy folk – not bad, considering the gradual demise of many churches throughout the UK. Today it's Reverend Brown's turn at the Church of Scotland for morning service. Evening service will be in the Methodist chapel, where Mr James Wilson, a lay preacher, and Annie's brother, is in charge.

I hurry along with the wind and the sleet for company. Then I hear it, the church bells ringing. I love those bells as they remind me that Fair Isle, small as it is, keeps up the old traditions. There's something comforting about that sound.

Georgie is the bell ringer. With yellow oilskins gone, a navy-blue suit, crisp white shirt and tie, he's metamorphosed into a church elder.

Then I remember Tommy saying, 'It's a peerie place and we all lend a hand at whatever needs doing.'

Since my arrival I've never missed a Sunday service, and if I had missed one for no good reason it would certainly be frowned on. Such is the way of the isle on Sunday. No maakin, no radio, no washing of clothes, and the bare necessities when it comes to cooking. It's not a surprise. I grew up with these same doctrines of keeping the Sabbath holy. But after a few years of London in the sixties, it now seems quaint and old-fashioned. I'm determined, though, to integrate myself into island ways, and I begin to find this routine refreshing and very good for the soul. Our spiritual lives are indeed well catered for in Fair Isle.

I'm no sooner back home from church when a pretty young girl knocks urgently on my door. I recognise her as one of the volunteers sent to Fair Isle by the National Trust for Scotland to help renovate houses, dig tracks and generally keep the island well maintained.

'I'm so sorry to interrupt you. I'm Kirsten and I'm very worried about Brendan, one of our colleagues. He's not at all well and in a lot of pain.'

'I'll come back with you, Kirsten.' I try hard to reassure this white-faced, anxious girl. 'I'll have a look at Brendan and then we'll take it from there.'

Despite the bedroom being cold, Brendan's face is flushed and he's sweating profusely, 'I've never experienced pain like this.' He reaches out desperately for my hand. 'I'm sorry to have called you out on a Sunday.'

'That's what I'm here for, I can see you're suffering.' I sit by his bed and try to comfort him. Here's this young lad, completely out of his comfort zone and no doubt full of worry about what chance there is of medical help on this isolated island. 'I'm right here, Brendan, please don't worry. We'll get you to a hospital if that's what's needed.'

A shadow of relief crosses his face as I place the thermometer under his tongue and feel his abdomen. 'Gosh, Brendan, your temperature is over 100 degrees and your abdomen is like a board. It's appendicitis, I'm sure. As soon as I've contacted Dr Mainland, I'll be right back, I promise, and I'll have some strong painkillers for you.'

'Ah, thank you, Nurse, and could you please let my mum know?' I pat his shoulder and give him a reassuring smile. 'Of course I will. I see you live in Edinburgh. Try and relax if you can. I'll be back before you know it.'

'Hello there, Nurse, what can I do for you?' I'm sure I'm interrupting Dr Mainland's Sunday dinner

'It's one of the volunteers, Doctor. Brendan Scott. He's in a lot of pain, and I'm sure it's appendicitis.'

'Well, we'll not take any chances. Let's get him to the Gilbert Bain Hospital straight away.'

Fortunately, the weather is fair. The *Good Shepherd* is duly commissioned to take Brendan to Grutness. Administering a strong painkiller, I make him as comfortable as possible in a lower bunk. Pulling up a box to sit on, I settle down to observe my patient with every scrap of my attention. I have seen too many burst appendix cases to be complacent.

I am reminded of my first trip, when Alec held my head. Due to the painkiller, Brendan is fast asleep, so I hold his hand all the way to Grutness. Now and again he opens his eyes, gives a weak smile and squeezes my hand. Fortunately, he isn't seasick. Can't say the same about me. At least twice on the journey, the old National Dried Milk tin comes in handy. Da Roost doesn't get any better. I put the thought of the immediate return journey firmly out of my mind.

By the time we get to Grutness, I am feeling pretty ghastly. The ambulance is ready and waiting. I feel strange passing 'my' patient over to the ambulance driver, but he's more than competent. 'I'll look after him, Nurse, don't you worry. By the look of you, I think you could do well with a doctor yourself.'

'You cheeky thing,' I retort, waving the ambulance on its way.

Loyal Christine. 'You're an angel,' I tell her, when she insists that the crew and I stop over for a cup of tea, before tackling Da Roost once more.

After a restless night, I'm up bright and early, waiting anxiously to hear the outcome of Brendan's illness.

Eventually, Dr Mainland's call comes through. 'It wasn't appendicitis, after all.' The sense of failure hits me right in the solar plexus. I was so sure, and I was so wrong. Oh no, he's going to lose all confidence in me.

He tells me that Brendan is still in hospital undergoing observation and tests. 'He's in a lot of pain. They're querying diverticulitis or colitis. The symptoms of these conditions are often suggestive of appendicitis, as you know. Time will tell.'

'Thanks for the call,' I replied shakily, 'I do feel a bit better that my diagnosis and transfer wasn't a total blunder.'

'Not at all,' Dr Mainland reassures me. 'Far better to err on the side of caution and, in any case, he did need hospitalisation. I've just spoken to his family in Edinburgh and they're relieved that Brendan is being looked after.'

CHAPTER 11

I'm far too young for this job, too inexperienced, too sensitive. I catch myself at it again, and detect moistness around my eyes. I pull sharply and give myself a good lecture. I really must stop mulling over mistakes. Come to think of it, I shouldn't view it as a mistake at all. Brendan is far better off in hospital and I'm doing my best. Then I find myself chuckling when I tell myself, 'At least you haven't killed anyone … yet!' No sooner have I finished lecturing myself than I'm back to beating myself up.

My thoughts and ponderings are not doing me any good. I do a quick Monday round, telling folks I'll come again tomorrow, with the excuse that I'm tired after the *Good Shepherd* trip. The best thing I can do is go to my favourite spot.

It's a dreich day, but I'm determined. I clearly remember dad's words, 'Where's your backbone, lass?' I shake myself out of self-pity. It's 1.30pm. I'd better hurry, otherwise the darkness will put a stop to my walk. I pull on a pair of wellington boots and, trying hard to ignore the wind and the sleet, I set out for Malcolm's Head. I'm glad of my waterproof jacket to keep me cosy and dry. Battling the elements, I note there are no rabbits or bonnie flowers to vie for my attention this time round. Even my dear pals, the Tammie Norries, are long gone, somewhere out to sea.

The inky storm clouds are hanging low over a slate sea. I deliberately stop myself from thinking that this scene is reflecting my mood. Instead, I give myself permission to confront my thoughts. I have always had someone in my life in whom I can confide, and to whom I can vent my feelings, without being judged.

I am homesick. Now the realisation is out, at least inside my head. I miss the city life and the excitement. I miss having a female friend. I miss having a confidante. I thought I was a country girl, but maybe I'm not?

I waste no time. I make my way back across the sleety cliff tops, skirting water holes and boggy patches. I take a moment or two to admire 'Queen Victoria', then a vision of a bath takes over and I hurry on home. There, I learn that Dr Mainland has phoned. Brendan does indeed have colitis, and is now receiving the treatment he needs.

Hot, relaxing baths always do the trick. I try not to think about what I still see as my failure, nor my homesickness, but focus instead on the coming week's itinerary. Tomorrow – Tuesday – I'll visit as many households as possible. I enjoy these visits immensely and they give me a chance to ensure that the elderly residents of the isle, particularly, are having their needs met. The thought gives me comfort.

CHAPTER 12

My first visit, this cold foggy morning, is to the shop. The fog horns are groaning from both lighthouses. Two blasts from the South Lighthouse, three from the North. Thank goodness for lighthouses. Before they were built in Fair Isle, many ships and boats met their end on the treacherous rocks.

The *Good Shepherd* does a twice-weekly routine trip to the Shetland mainland, on Tuesday and Friday, bringing goods to the local shop. Stewart and Sheila Wilson run a lively shop, a meeting place for the Fair Isle folks. Long chats and catching up are the order of the day, especially on Wednesday and Saturday when goods such as bread are still fresh.

My visits to the shop are many. Sometimes, as the nurse, I keep my eye on Sheila and her pregnancy, but on other occasions I visit as a customer. The Wilsons are young and innovative and keep up to date with what's new in the retail world, and strive to bring in cost-effective as well as nourishing products. Oranges and apples and bananas are plentiful as are dried fruit and nuts.

Sheila takes an interest in all aspects of her pregnancy, and will make sure that the latest in the way of baby and pregnancy magazines are always at hand. She's certainly on the ball, and will often challenge me with her knowledge. This morning is no different. 'Would you please give me a few childbirth education classes and teach me the best way to breathe when I'm in labour?'

'Of course, Sheila,' I exclaim. 'How about tomorrow? I'll come after tea, about seven? Make sure Stewart is with you when I show off my wisdom.' We both laugh.

'Thanks, Nurse, see you tomorrow.'

My next visit is to Edith and Jimmy Stout, who live across the road from my house. They are kindness itself. I often have a leg of lamb for my Sunday roast thrust into my hands, along with a dozen eggs and an invitation for tea, all of which has made me feel at home. The Stouts have five children. Four have flown the nest – Jimmy, the eldest, is at agricultural college in Aberdeenshire, Teddy is training to be a ship's officer in the merchant navy, then Edith Ann and Andrew are at the Anderson Institute in Lerwick. Maurice, the baby of the family, lives at home

We settle down beside the warm fire. Midway is a happy, homely house. The many smiling faces in the photographs on the mantelpiece are evidence of a close, loving family. The organ, standing proudly against the wall, is the first thing I notice when I enter. Edith is the church organist and, whenever I visit, I ask her to play. She's a talented and sensitive musician who loves to play. The lovely strains of a favourite hymn do me good and cheer me up considerably, especially when, through the window, I notice the fog threatening to obliterate the whole isle.

Edith tells me news about her children, who all write extremely welcome letters. Although I have never met them, I feel that I already know them. 'They'll soon be home for Christmas,' Edith can't hide her excitement.

After a while, Jimmy joins us. He has a great sense of humour and is full of jokes. A hard worker, he takes pride in his croft and also takes his turn as skipper on the *Good Shepherd*.

It would be lovely just to sit here in this cosy kitchen for the rest of the day, but duty calls. After a good half-hour of banter and chat, it's time for my next visit. Jimmy comes to the door with me.

'Now, Nurse Mona, it's such a shame you have to be out and about in this weather, but tell me, how are you doing?' I have this conversation with Jimmy every week. He's a caring man and I know he's genuinely interested. This is not just small talk.

'I'm doing fine. I'm gradually getting to know the folks and gaining their confidence, I hope.' Then that all-too-familiar lump rises in my throat. I swallow hard before replying. 'No, I'm telling you fibs, Jimmy, I'm sorry. I've been feeling a bit down in the dumps of late, thinking about all the things I miss. I miss mam and dad and the family. Then there's all the mistakes just waiting to happen. I ken I'm probably a bit hard on mesel.'

'I do understand, my lass. It can't be easy for you. We're isolated here. Maybe the day will come when we'll get a plane, maybe even a helicopter. Imagine that now. I suppose it's a bit of a pipe dream, but the wye the world is going, you never do know.' He puts a fatherly hand on my shoulder and goes on to reassure me, and remind me that Christmas is around the corner. 'Wir bairns will be hame, what you need is some fun. Just you wait 'til we have wir Christmas party.'

The rest of the day is spent popping into houses along the way. No, pop is not the right word. I grope my way along the road, cross stiles and tackle muddy fields. The fog gets thicker, with no sign of a let-up. I blunder along, literally feeling my way. Then, thank goodness, Busta looms out of the mist and at last I know where I am.

In every house I visit I'm made to feel welcome, with offers of food and warm beverages. To refuse these offers would be considered rude, so I do the best I can, reminding myself that, if this carries on, I will be as fat as a selkie before long.

I'm pleased to hear there are no major problems. On my rounds, I dispense chronic medications, check blood pressures and make appointments. I realise that I am enjoying district nursing, as most of my nursing duties are house calls. My clinic caters for the well and healthy, along with those with minor ailments. Cuts and bruises, suturing of wounds, changes of dressings, injections and immunisations are done in the clinic. I don't have set times to work. I'm on call 24 hours, and I make appointments as needed.

As I make my rounds the thought occurs to me that, on the whole, the Fair Isle folks are a healthy lot, both physically and mentally, and I ask myself why. It strikes me that, along with hard work and exercise, there's very little in the way of alcohol consumption. It's all clean living and a mostly organic diet. Could that be it? Oh, yes, and I mustn't forget, strong spiritual faith. This is all very different from what I was used to in the casualty and out-patient departments of the big hospitals down south, where the use of drugs and alcohol were far too prevalent, along with violence and abuse of women and children.

Well, one thing I must confess: this life I'm living here in Fair Isle gives me time to think, time to imagine and time for my very favourite hobby of writing. Yet another thought crosses my mind – preoccupied as I am with finding my way through the wet, cold fog, it's a miracle I can even think, never mind day-dream – I tell myself that, if ever the opportunity should arise, I will research the way of life and its influence on health in the remote islands of Scotland, and then write a thesis. Ah, Mona – I feel my lips turn up at the corners, and chide myself gently – pigs might fly. Stop dreaming, girl.

Now it's Helen and Lottie's turn. I visit Ootra every Monday afternoon. Helen is a widow, having lost her husband when he fell over the cliffs. Lottie is a spinster and dependent on Helen, her stronger, younger sister. They are very lovable and I enjoy our conversations, which frequently carry us back to their childhoods. I have a great interest in family history, so I listen intently to their stories about what life was like in Fair Isle when they were little girls.

Today, as always, Helen begins, 'It wasn't easy back when we were peerie. Folk struggled just to keep going. Back then, the whole isle belonged to the laird. Oh, the lairds, they didn't care, and would have chased the crofters aff their bits of crofts if they couldn't come up with the rent. We were lucky, I suppose, as father ran the post office and the phone exchange, so we never had to worry about whar wir money cam fae.'

As she pauses, Lottie repeats her last sentence, 'So we never had to worry about whar wir money cam fae.'

I never tire of their stories and, as the months go on, I'm sure they'll help me piece together the history of Fair Isle.

Both sisters are sticklers for time. A grand, old clock is their reference point. From my first visit to Ootra, it became clear that they want my visit to start at four and end at five, when they have their tea. 'So, we'll see you at four next Monday, and then you'll be ready to go home for your tea.

Helen and Lottie always 'dress up' for my visit. They wear nice frocks and cardigans. I do feel honoured that they show their respect for me in this way. I make a point of admiring their gold brooches and real pearl necklaces.

'Thank you, Nurse, this one belonged to mother, and this one to grandmother,' says Helen. A silver-plated tray with a crystal sherry glass is always ready and waiting. 'You'll tak a peerie corn o' sherry, Nurse. You've had a long walk and it'll warm you up.'

Lottie echoes her, as she always does, 'You've had a long walk and it'll warm you up.'

Two doors up from Ootra lives Willie Eunson. When describing

48

people, the Fair Isle folk always preface their name with the house they live in. Willie Eunson is known as Leogh Willie. Leogh is a typical, old-fashioned 'but and ben' Shetland cottage, spartan and clean.

Willie is elderly and lives alone. I like to think that he enjoys my Monday visit. Strongly independent, Willie looks after himself well, despite having only one functioning arm. He told me he had an illness when he was very young that left his arm useless. At first, he was a bit sceptical about my nursing prowess and, still now, can't resist testing me on my abilities on many fronts. 'Du's brawly young, is du no?' I smile, but say nothing. 'Can du milk a coo? And whit aboot maetin da hens, is du a dab hand at dat?'

'Yes, Willie I can do dat, no bother.'

'I'm blyde tae hear dat. Sometimes in da winter we are aa laid low we da flu, maybe du'll be da onyeen standin.'

I sincerely hope it will never come to that. 'I'm a Shetland lass, Willie,' I tell him, 'And things ir no dat much different here.'

'Am I no blyde tae hae a Shetland nurse. Dis nurses fae sooth nedder ken whit I'm sayin tae dem and I hiv no idea whit dey ir sayin tae me.' A back-handed compliment if ever I heard one

Willie is well read and clever. I know he understands far more than he lets on. We are never at a loss for conversation, discussing the daily news and politics. My visits to him keep me on my toes.

I'm tired when I get home. I promise myself I'll write my nursing notes first thing in the morning. There's nothing like fresh air – even foggy air – and exercise to encourage a deep, refreshing sleep.

Wednesday at 7.00pm I'm dressed in a tracksuit and I'm off to the shop, armed with colourful graphs, a plastic female pelvis, a doll with a good hard head and a soft cloth body, complete with belly button to which is attached an umbilical cord and a placenta. I laugh at the memory of my training days. Our class of pupil midwives each carefully pleated our own baby cord, made from red and blue wool, then carefully knitted and felted the dark red placenta. Little did I think then that this work of art, or more accurately, this monstrosity, would land up in Fair Isle.

Sheila and Stewart are ideal pupils, interested and curious, and they ask non-stop questions. 'Show us again how the baby will come through the pelvis?' asks Sheila.

Stewart, not to be outdone, asks, 'My goodness, is the cord that long?'

'Yes, it is,' I say. 'The cord is the life-line between mother and the unborn baby. See here, the blue thread depicts the umbilical vein that carries oxygen and nutrients from mum's placenta to baby, then the two red threads are the umbilical arteries. They carry the deoxygenated blood and waste products, such as carbon dioxide, back to mum's placenta.'

Stewart's eyes widen. 'As the Good Book tells us, we truly are fearfully and wonderfully made.'

'You're right, Stewart. I hope you'll be with Sheila when baby's born. I've delivered quite a number of babies and, each time I do, I hold my own breath until baby takes its first breath. The miracle of childbirth – I never tire of watching it unfold.'

'He'll be there, alright,' says Sheila.

'I wouldn't miss it for the world,' says Stewart. And I think I even detect a tear in his eye.

'When you're in the early stages of labour, don't lie down. Keep upright and keep walking. Breathe slowly and try and relax if you can. That goes for you too, Stewart.'

'I've been reading in the pregnancy and baby magazines that relaxing in warm water can help?' Sheila asks.

'It certainly can. Stewart can hold your hand and help you breathe. Just follow your body's instincts, and your midwife will keep you both right.'

'I'll just think about the Johnny Walker ad, "Keep Walking",' says Stewart, and laughs heartily.

I keep my childbirth education class light and informative and am rewarded with many questions, as well as many laughs. Both Sheila and Stewart tell me they have thoroughly enjoyed themselves and look forward to the next class.

CHAPTER 13

The phone is ringing when I get home. It's 10.00pm and I feel a twinge of anxiety, thinking this might well be an emergency.

It's my mother. 'Is everything all right, Mam?' I blurt out, feeling somewhat uneasy. It's not like mam to phone at this hour.

'Dad and I are missing you so much, we've decided to come and see you and have a bit of a holiday.' My anxiety turns to excitement. I tell mam that I can't wait to see them. 'We'll be in next Tuesday. Dad says it's not the best time of year, but he misses you too.'

Then I remember Da Roost. How will they contend with that demon? Mam reassures me that she's never been seasick. 'Dad is not such a good sailor, so I'm planning to fill him full of seasickness tablets.' We both laugh. 'He's all for it, so keen to see you, and see Fair Isle. It's been a dream of his for a while so, if you're for it, and have a bed for us, we'll come next week.'

I'm thrilled with the news and put aside concerns about the journey. They're getting on in years, but then they've had plenty of experience of the vagaries of the sea. I'd better get cracking and make my house sparkle. I only have a week.

I can hardly contain myself when the *Good Shepherd* comes into view. I really do have a love/hate relationship with my lifeline. Oh, old tub, I'm thinking, I need you, but you really do make me sick. Then I see them: mam, with her big broad smile, and dad looking exactly how I felt after a bad *Good Shepherd* journey.

I'm crying, they're laughing, we're hugging and we're all speaking at once. Bystanders look at us with knowing smiles and give us a thumbs-up. We make our way up the track to where Stewart's van is ready and waiting to take us home. Stewart heaves the suitcases into the back of the van and the four of us squeeze into the front as best we can.

The wind is definitely on the rise. Dad tells me the *Good Shepherd* took a hammering from the merciless waves, but plays down his seasickness. 'I ken all about the sea and it's not the first time I've felt the effects of her. I recover fast, don't you worry.'

Stewart's van is now taking a hammering from the wind and the rain, so we don't loiter to show my parents the Sheep Rock or other scenic treasures. The goal is to get home as fast as Stewart can manoeuvre his trusty van through the storm.

We're windswept and wet by the time we get to my house. I am glad I have the place warm and welcoming for my dear mam and dad. The old Rayburn is hiding our dinner. Cooking is another talent that I don't possess. Having spent all my training years in nurses' homes, we nurses just ate what was set before us. Sometimes it was okay and, at other times, horrendous. But we never learned to do any better ourselves, more's the pity.

Since arriving in Fair Isle, I've been spoilt for choice. Many invitations for lunch and dinner have let me off the hook, but I had to do something with the fish, chicken, the lamb roasts, and the tasty home-grown vegetables I've been so generously offered. I've been scouring recipe books, writing down instructions from the Fair Isle housewives, and now I'm hoping my parents will be surprised by my new skill.

I usually eat in the kitchen but today, to celebrate, the open fire is glowing in the sitting room and, for the first time since my arrival, I've set up the dining table with a cloth and my 'best' crockery and cutlery, courtesy of the Zetland County Council.

Afterwards, we sit back in comfy chairs and, despite the fact that the house is shaking with the force of the wind, I'm feeling proud of myself as I hear their compliments about my Yorkshire pudding and tasty gravy. It's great to hear the home news first-hand. We spend a good few hours catching up, but I'm conscious of the generator clicking off at 11.00pm so I've made hot water bottles and candles ready.

'I'm so vexed the weather's turned bad,' I say, with disappointment in my voice. 'I had all kinds of walks planned so that you could see the isle. I'm glad I did all my visits yesterday. We'll just have to hunker down till things improve. If I'm needed, someone will come for me.'

I'm reassured that their visit is to see me. They are quite happy to rest and relax, and if and when the weather gets better we'll take it from there. As it is, we are snug and cosy in our beds long before the generator clicks off.

I don't sleep well. The howling and banging of the wind makes me uneasy. I'm familiar with bad weather but this sounds serious. My bedside clock reads 3.15am when I'm woken by an especially loud noise. I light the small paraffin lamp and get up.

I meet mam in the doorway. 'Sounds kinda ominous,' she says. 'I've been awake since two o'clock. Dad, of course, can sleep through anything. I hope the Fair Isle folk have battened down the hatches.'

We check doors and windows and all seems fine. I'm guessing this house has seen many a storm. I tell mam that I am so blyde her and dad are here. 'It's a bit scary all on my own.'

Mam comes up with her cure-all – a cup of tea. We stir up the

54

Rayburn and, in no time, we're sitting chatting while all hell has been let loose outside.

For the next two days the storm, if anything, gets worse. Dad is an expert at reading my wall barometer and he listens faithfully to the shipping forecast on my tiny portable radio. More childhood memories come flooding back as I hear, 'Tyne, Dogger, Fastnet, Lundy, Rockall, Bailey'. Back in the day, before TV, most Shetland households listened in religiously every morning and evening but I had all but forgotten the shipping forecast. Then, there it is – 'Fair Isle'. We stay dead quiet as the cultured, cut-glass BBC voice tells us, 'Gale force 8, reaching storm force 11. High seas and heavy rains to continue.'

The *Good Shepherd* will not start out in wind force 7, so there's no hope that Friday's journey will take place. Mam and dad have brought in lots of my favourite goodies. They both laugh when I say, 'At least we'll not starve, and bang goes my diet.'

Dad is a ferocious reader so this enforced confinement is right up his street. Mam has taken it upon herself to teach me a few baking tricks and, when we're not baking, we play board games and catch up on family goings-on. Time does not lie heavy on our hands.

It's tea-time on Thursday when I hear the loud banging on my door. At first I think it's the wind but, when I open up, I see a very wet Tommy, looking as if he has just stepped out of the sea.

CHAPTER 14

'Come in, Tommy,' I say tentatively. I'm convinced that, in this weather, this isn't just a social visit.

Tommy's strong features register concern as he says, 'We were concerned about Uncle Willum, Auntie Jean and Auntie Bab. It's some hike fae Busta tae Lower Staneybrake whar dey bide, but we could'na settle 'til we were sure they were alright.'

This is typical of Fair Isle living. The close community looks after each other, so there's no need for me to worry about someone falling ill without it being brought to my notice.

I visit Lower Staneybrake regularly. Willum and Bab, although well past middle age, are strong and healthy. But Jean, Willum's wife and Bab's sister, is failing. On my last visit I noted that she was looking a bit fragile. She brushed my concerns aside, but now it seems they were justified.

'You'll need to come and see her, Nurse, she's not well. Uncle tells me she coughed most of the night and she can't get out of her bed today.'

I'm convinced that if Tommy weren't holding on tightly to my arm

I'd blow clean away. The icy rain is pelting my face and the wind is ferocious as we both lean into it. Staneybrake is not far from my house so after about 20 minutes we're there.

Jean's temperature is sky-high, she's shivery and is feeling dreadful. She is also delirious. Her cough is rasping and, when I listen in to her chest, I realise it's definitely a chest infection, maybe even bronchitis. No X-ray department in Fair Isle to help you, Mona, I'm thinking. I trust that it's not pneumonia.

The family are obviously concerned. I tell them that, as soon as I've had a word with Dr Mainland, I'll be back. Nurses say the most ridiculous things sometimes. 'Now, don't you worry,' is but one. It's the best I can do, as Tommy and I once again face the great outdoors.

CHAPTER 15

Dr Mainland and I have a long chat. I tell him that Jean's throat and ears appear normal, the problem lies on her chest. I boldly tell him that I think its bronchitis. I dare not even voice the word pneumonia.

I detect a note of anxiety in Dr Mainland's voice. 'She's obviously very ill. She's 73, you say? Not a good scenario and, in this weather, there's no chance of a transfer to hospital.'

As Dr Mainland speaks, I'm thinking fast. I'm silent for about five seconds before I suggest that, whatever happens with the weather, we keep the old lady in Fair Isle. I'll follow whatever treatment he orders, and I'll nurse her. 'Even in the best of weather, I doubt she would make the journey, frail as she is.'

'By what you're telling me, she might not survive this illness. Be it bronchitis ... or even pneumonia.' There, he's said it. After giving it time to sink in, he goes on. 'What does matter is, will you be able to manage?'

'I'm sure I will,' I say firmly. 'There are plenty of relatives around to help.' Dr Mainland goes on to give me strict instructions, and I promise I'll phone immediately if I need more advice. While I'm preparing my medical bag, Tommy is conversing with my parents. He has a strong, loud voice so I can hear every word. Now it's his turn to tell them not to worry about me and to reassure them that he'll be by my side until Auntie Jean and the household has settled.

I shout back from the clinic room, 'I won't be home tonight. I'm going to stay until I see how it goes.'

If anything, the weather conditions are still worsening. Tommy and I struggle back to Lower Staneybrake. Tommy's huge torch has little effect against the wrath of the storm. 'Haad du on to me, and pit dy head doon and face her straight on.'

I obey without question. Step by step we make it back. With a sense of relief, our sodden rain clothes are discarded in the back porch and we replace them with warm woollens; Tommy thinks of everything. Then we set about calming the storm inside.

First, we make sure that Uncle Willum is comfortable by the kitchen fire. Willum is the man responsible for making the island's coffins. I'm wondering if he's thinking that his next assignment will be for his dear wife.

I hijack Bab to be my nursing assistant. To nurse Jean we've decided to keep her in the 'ben end'. Ben is the best room in the house. It's airy and spacious and has an open fireplace. Tommy and Bab set up a single comfortable bed. I'm happy with this as it makes care and nursing so much easier.

Bab is a strong woman with a gentle voice. She tenderly helps me wash and dress Jean, and is quick on the uptake when I explain the method of changing an ill person's bedding. 'Du's doing great, Bab. I'm grateful du's here to help, I tell her.

'I'll try my best, as lang as du gives me instructions.'

At last, we have Jean propped up on pillows to ease her breathing. The tick-tock of the clock on the mantle shelf and the comforting hiss of the lamp has a soothing effect on both of us.

I prop a pillow behind Bab's head. 'You've done a great job, Auntie Bab, tak a rest now.'

Bab gives a sigh and a smile and sits by the bed holding her sister's hand, while I get going with the observations and medications.

Jean is very ill. Her eyes plead with me when I encourage sips of water from a teaspoon. 'Jean, maybe du could try a peerie sip of water?'

There's no response. I gently rub her parched lips with glycerine and abandon trying to administer medication by mouth. I hate having to inflict pain, especially on the elderly, but I have to resort to intra-muscular injections.

'I'm so sorry, Jean,' I whisper in her ear. 'This is going to hurt a peerie bit.' Jean's breathing is very shallow but the coughing has stopped. She simply hasn't the strength to cough. I visualise the mucous and gunk lying there in her chest and pray the antibiotics will soon take effect.

Tommy insists that he must go to Busta as his parents will be worried. 'I'll be back, I certainly won't leave you here. Anything might happen and, with no phone, you'll be stuck.'

I tell him I'm forever grateful. It's a trek to Busta, but he's a strong man, both in voice and body. How he managed to help me keep my feet on the road, I'll never know.

It's been a challenging day for both Bab and Willum and I encourage them to get a good night's sleep. 'It will be a busy day for us all tomorrow. It's important you rest. I'm right here with Jean. Tommy will soon be back to keep me company.' I paste a smile on my face, hoping that will allay their fears.

By the time Tommy is back, with yet another change of clothes tied up in a plastic bag, I'm enjoying a rest and downing my third cup of coffee. From the noises emerging from both their bedrooms, I know Bab and Willum are asleep.

60

I encourage Tommy to make up a bed on the kitchen couch. 'I'll be fine, I really will, and I promise to give you a shout if I need you. I'm on high alert. Night duty is nothing new for me.'

It's a long night. I keep myself going with cups of coffee, attending to the fire and the lamp ... The lamp, yes. I can't help but think of myself as a bit of a Florence Nightingale. I chuckle. I'm thrilled to find a *People's Friend* magazine to keep me awake and interested.

Four in the morning is the crucial hour. Nurses the world over will confirm that this is when the patient will be at her most vulnerable. The darkest hour is just before dawn. I wonder if that's how the saying came about. It's around this time that I become convinced Jean has passed on. She's deathly still and quiet. I listen in ... and hear her heart, but the beat is slow. I give her a little shake and tell her she's doing great. Good, there's a flicker of her eyelids. She opens her eyes briefly and stares at me blankly.

It takes me half-an-hour to get Jean to sip two tablespoons of water. She's very dehydrated and I have to be patient. 'You're doing great, Auntie Jean. That's it, another peerie sip.'

Next, it's another injection. She gives a moan and I feel very cruel. But needs must. I gently roll her over and change her position before attempting the next spoons of water. She is a little stronger and seems thirsty. I'm cheered.

It's 7.30am. My nose must be deceiving me. The smell of toast and coffee envelops me like a caress. And there stands my knight in shining oilskins. 'Oh, Tommy, toast and coffee, what would I do without you?' We both tuck into this early breakfast before thinking up a plan for the day.

The next three days pass in a blur. I stay with Jean until midday. She is still very ill. Once I've made her comfortable and given her her medication, I leave her in the care of Bab.

Tommy is happy with the arrangement. 'Uncle is fairly fit, I know, but it's not fair to expect him to come fur dee if needed. This storm is not easing, so I'll just bide and give Auntie Bab a hand.

I'm relieved. 'That's good of you, Tommy. I'll sleep in peace knowing you're here. I'll be back at eight to do night shift.'

It's a relief to go home and be pampered by mam. I'm so pleased my folks are with me. 'Seems we got here in the nick of time,' says mam, philosophically. 'Now make sure du has a good sleep. Annie and Stewart have been alang, and they tell us the whole isle knows what's going on. Not to worry, everybody is looking out for each other. This too shall pass. Young Stewart is going to tak dee back to Lower Staneybrake, he'll lat Tommy ken.'

By the third day I detect a slight improvement in Jean. I phone Dr Mainland to give him an update. 'I hope it's not just my wishful thinking, Doctor, but her pulse is stronger, her temperature is normal and she's more aware.'

'That is encouraging, to say the least. How's the fluid intake?'

'She's drinking, small sips still. She loves sweet tea and I'm hoping that will keep her blood sugar level up.'

'Good news, Nurse, dehydration has to be avoided.'

'I'm hoping, if she improves, I'll be able to give meds by mouth. The whole isle has rallied to the cause and I have offers of help from all quarters.'

'You're doing a good job. Keep up the good work and, remember, give me a call any time if you need to chat.'

It's a week since mam and dad arrived in Fair Isle and much has happened in that time. Today's Tuesday. I wonder if there's any chance of the *Good Shepherd* making the crossing to Grutness. I get edgy when we're cut off and have grave doubts about my ability if truly challenged. To my ears there is no easing of the wind. This is confirmed when I hear the weatherman say, 'Wind now at gale force 7.'

Mam is busy preparing my dinner to 'keep your strength up' (lamb chops and new tatties – great), when dad quietly enters the clinic room where I'm busy repacking and replacing Jean's meds.

'Mam and I have had a long chat and we've decided that we're going to bide wi dee until Christmas. If this weather does ease up, the *Good Shepherd* will get back to normal and, mind, the bairns are due hame from the Anderson Institute for their holidays and if Jean continues to improve the isle will have plenty to celebrate. We might even see a bit, oot and aboot, afore we go back.'

I tell my father that I'm so glad to have him and mam here. I can't emphasise this enough. 'But Dad, we mustn't count our chickens. Jean is a very old and a very ill woman, anything could happen. Christmas might well be a very sad time. A funeral, maybe.'

'Lass, does du no think we've thought about dat?' Hang in dere. So far, so good, and it's aye good to remain positive.'

CHAPTER 16

Some would thank their lucky stars, others providence, maybe. Not me. I remember my prayer that first day in Fair Isle and I thank the Lord for seeing me through three hard weeks. All glory to Him and to my small army of helpers. I could not have done without Him or them.

It's nearing Christmas, the Fair Isle big bairns are home, and the peerie ones are also on school holiday. But for me, Auntie Jean is still my concern. I've got so used to hearing them referring to each other as Auntie Jean, Auntie Bab, and Uncle Willum, that I've started addressing them in the same way, not even aware that I'm doing it. I apologise, but the relatives who matter think it's charming.

Auntie Jean is certainly a soldier. I keep reminding myself that she's far from out of the woods. On the bright side, she has responded to the medications and, although weak and *very* frail, she can now take a little clear soup and warm milk, but still gets fed up with the water I insist she drinks. Her voice is scarcely audible, but she can whisper 'yes' and 'no', and can shake her head to my queries.

During her delirious episodes, thankfully now over, I worried in case her bright, intelligent brain would succumb to dementia but, no, her mental capacity seems intact.

I now visit Jean three times each day, then leave her in the care of friends and relatives. The weather has softened and, although it's still cold, I decide it's time to take my parents on a tour of the isle. This plan serves two purposes. Firstly, I'll be visiting each household, making sure that all are having their needs met. And, secondly, the isle folk are interested to meet mam and dad.

First visit is to my prime patient, Auntie Jean. Mam and dad have heard so much about her, they're a bit nervous at first, knowing how ill she's been. 'Do you think she'll be up for this?' asks dad.

'The only way to find out is to go,' I reply.

I have already dressed Jean in a brand-new frilly nightie that Auntie Bab found tucked away amongst Jean's best clothes. 'We really are a daft lot,' says Bab. 'Why on earth do we keep the best of things until, very often, it's too late to enjoy them.'

Bab is a wise woman. We agree that the two of us will not hoard a thing, and we'll enjoy and use everything while the going is good. It's a relief to have a peerie chuckle. I've also braided Jean's hair and held a mirror for her to see herself. She keeps tapping on her nightie, and I do detect a smile.

My parents are tender and loving with Jean. They are rewarded with whispers and head nods. We don't stay long. Auntie Jean always squeezes my hand very gently when I come and when I go. These small acts are not lost on my parents. Once outside, mam gives me a hug and dad pats my shoulder. No need for words.

Dad is keen to visit the bird observatory near North Haven. It's a pleasant walk. 'That's Upper Staneybrake, where Georgie and his father Dodie live. And this here is Barkland, Alec and Margaret's place.'

No sooner have I said the words than two blond boys come running to meet us. 'Michael and Kenneth, meet my mam and dad. We'd love you to join us on our walk.' I know these two lads well, having treated them for minor ailments in the clinic. They are bright wee boys and certainly not shy. They keep up a running commentary about their hopes for a bumper Christmas.

After a while they are ready to turn back. Mam is charmed by the little Vikings, as she calls them. 'We will come alang and visit if we have time. We met your dad Alec on the *Good Shepherd*, and we look forward to meeting your mam.'

It's so good to be out in the fresh air. We take our time and amble along, talking and laughing and joking. I feel blessed to have mam and dad all to myself. Being one of five children, I always had to share them. I grin at the thought and give myself a mental hug.

'That's Setter, there on the left.' I go on to tell them about Gordon Barnes, a young Englishman who got tired of life in the south and decided to transfer to Fair Isle. 'He rents Setter croft, and not only did he bring his farming skills, but he brought the first tractor to the isle.' Dad is impressed.

'He's been here since 1960 and, hopefully, he's committed to bide.' We discuss Gordon for a bit and I add, 'He's such a boon to the isle, helping out with land work, digging ditches and assisting with the modernisation of houses and crofts.'

We arrive at the bird observatory to be greeted by the warden, Roy Dennis. From what I'm told, Roy is an ornithologist of note. His love is the conservation of wild birds. The observatory is not a very attractive building, consisting of five Nissen huts – large prefabricated buildings with corrugated iron roofs – built in the last war and used by the Royal Navy.

Roy shows us around. He tells us that the observatory is really well-past its sell-by date, and he's hoping that in the not-too-distant future there will be funds available to build a state-of-the-art facility. He goes on to tell us a little about its history.

It seems Fair Isle saw a population low-point in the late 1940s, when there were only about 50 people left on the isle, and evacuation seemed a real possibility. This was avoided by George Waterston, a keen ornithologist who knew the isle was a stop-off point for many migrating birds. With the idea of using that fact to attract bird watchers, he bought the isle in 1948 and founded the Fair Isle Bird Observatory.

Roy's face takes on a look of excitement, mixed with a little pride, as he goes on. 'We can now claim to be the best place in Britain to spot rare birds. This brings in tourists and ornithologists from all over the world.' Roy smiles and turns to me. 'I know you've had a few at your door, Nurse, with cuts and bruises.'

I nod and tell him I'm pleased there hasn't been anything worse than that to treat.

Roy takes up his story again. 'The National Trust for Scotland soon saw the value of Fair Isle and bought the isle from George Waterston in 1955, and the rest is history.'

Roy is willing to show us around and I can see dad is taken with the room in which birds are ringed.

'I have plenty to take up my time here. What with monitoring migration and ringing the birds, my day flies past. Oops,' he laughs, 'pardon the pun.'

CHAPTER 17

Taking our leave from the observatory, we decide that's enough for one day, and walk slowly home. The wind has died down, the fog has lifted and there's a touch of frost in the air.

'This feels like Christmas,' says mam. 'Only three days to go. I've ordered a turkey to come in on Friday's *Good Shepherd*, that's if the wind is favourable. With a bit of luck, we'll have a traditional dinner on Saturday.'

While my life has been taken up with Auntie Jean and my parents, unbeknown to me great preparations have been going on for the Christmas party. Today, Annie tells me the village hall has been trans-formed. 'Oh, Mona, du'll love it. Just wait till du sees the balloons, the Christmas decorations and crackers. It's all set and ready to make this year's party the best yet.'

Normally, I would have been right in there helping out, but because my duty lies with Auntie Jean I have been excused. I'm tempted to take mam and dad along for a look, but we've decided to wait for the surprise.

When young Stewart brings the turkey along on Christmas Eve the conversation gets around to the party. 'I collected the tree aff the *Good Shepherd*,' Stewart is laughing. 'It's never Christmas withoot da tree, and a whole box of presents. The peerie wans are excited already. I've had a word with Dodie, he tells me that he has been commissioned to be Santie Klaas.'

Dad is now laughing. 'We'll never say a wird, Stewart, but tell wiz mair. Is there food and is there a dance?'

'Oh yes, indeed there is. I've been practising on my guitar already. My dad, of course, is a crack hand on the fiddle, and Alec plays the accordion. Neil is hame noo, and his love is also the guitar, so there is no excuse not tae dance.'

'My goodness me,' says mam. 'Your family are truly a talented lot, musicians as weel as spinning wheel makers and expert Fair Isle maakers.'

'Dad aye says the isle needs a time to dance and mak merry. A band is essential, so he made sure that if he couldn't find one, he would breed one, and so he did.' Now we're all laughing our heads off.

Mam makes busy preparing our Christmas dinner. It's a lovely moonlit night, and the stars are twinkling. Young Stewart has offered to walk with me to Lower Staneybrake. I sit with Jean every night as she still requires quite a bit of nursing care. I'm hoping that soon she'll be able to sleep through, but until such time I'll keep going. Stewart and I have become firm friends and enjoy each other's company. We have plenty to talk and laugh about tonight. On our way, we stare up at the clear bright sky. 'Maybe, if we're lucky, we'll see the aurora borealis,' he says.

'That wid truly be a treat, but as you ken, Stewart, the northern lights are unpredictable and full of surprises. If they decide not to show off, let's keep our eyes peeled for Santie's sledge. He'll be on his wye doon fae the North Pole.' The two of us are like bairns, remembering Christmases when we were peerie.

No sightings take place – of either Santie or the northern lights – but the sparkling frost on the ground, reflecting the waxing crescent moon and the twinkling stars, marks this as a Christmas Eve to remember.

Christmas morning, and a beautiful, crisp, frosty morning it is. I write a few lines in my diary. Saturday 25th December 1965. I'm thinking that this is one Christmas I'll never forget. After wishing Willum, Bab and Jean a happy Christmas, I make my way home and manage a few hours of sleep before our little family – me, mam and dad – open our presents, don our paper hats and pull crackers. My parents spoil me rotten and I am feeling very special and much loved.

The falling of the sun and the crisp, crunchy frost has bathed Fair Isle in a surreal light. After a sumptuous dinner, we take a stroll to Staneybrake. Mam has packed a basket with a full-on dinner and, while Auntie Bab and Uncle Willum tuck in, I make Jean comfortable, giving her a running commentary on my day so far. She's been living on semi-fluids, consistently refusing solid food. Perhaps because it's Christmas I decide, without expectation, to offer a peerie grain of mam's trifle. Her eyes light up and I am rewarded with a smile and a clear, 'Bless you.' It makes my day.

Willum, a quiet, unassuming man, has been a strong support for me during Jean's illness. He never fails to tell me how grateful he is for my efforts at keeping Jean comfortable. I note today there is a new light in his eyes at the prospect of his dear wife's recovery.

'It's early days, Willum, but the signs are good, so we keep hoping and praying that Auntie Jean will continue to improve.'

'We've been together for a mighty long time. She's my life, but I ken we are getting old and I have to be ready if she doesn't mak it.' Willum goes on to tell me about the coffin making. 'There are a few men on the isle that are good with woodwork, so we get together when needed.'

I'm finding this information fascinating. It appeals to my vivid imagination. The coffins are made from driftwood brought in by the sea. No fancy oak products with solid brass handles, just a simple box made with love, for a dear departed relative.

'Traditionally, Fair Isle men are beachcombers,' says Willum, 'or should I say cliff-combers. You'll have noticed the piles of sea treasures when you're on your rounds.'

'Yes, I have, Willum. All sorts of things: sea buoys and nets and, of course, lots of wood.'

'This goes back to when we had to rely on our wits to furnish our houses as well as make our coffins, so each and every bit of wood holds value. We all have a pile stacked up in our lofts.'

We turn our attention back to Jean. I'm comforted to see that she is relaxed and sleeping. 'I don't have to go to the party, Willum. I'll just bide here beside you.'

'You'll do no such thing. Bab and I will be fine and Tommy's promised to come back and fore to check up on wiz. Off you go and enjoy yourself. It will be ower by half-past-eleven, since it's Sunday tomorrow. I'll bide up until you come back for Jean, and I look forward to hearing all aboot it.'

It's 4.00pm by the time I get myself all dolled up for the party. It suddenly occurs to me that this is the first time in months that I've paid attention to my hair, or applied make-up. Then I scratch around for my favourite party dress. I nearly didn't pack it for Fair Isle, but now I'm happy I did and am surprised at myself for feeling excited. A far cry from my wild days in London, I'm thinking, when I danced the night away at the Hammersmith Odeon and Chelsea Town Hall. The Fair Isle village hall is exactly what I need tonight. I'm determined to enjoy myself.

CHAPTER 18

The hall is a spectacle, with the tree as its focal point, surrounded by lights and excited bairns. The tables are groaning with traditional shortbread, Annie's large Christmas cake, mince pies and bowls of oranges and apples – luxuries in Fair Isle. The atmosphere is relaxed and jovial and I'm glad to see mam and dad enjoying themselves. The Fair Isle folks have taken them to their hearts and are introducing them all around.

For myself, it's good to see new faces, mostly young faces at that. Edith and Jimmy's family are introduced and I'm immediately taken with their daughter, Edith Ann. She's interested in nursing and is full of questions about my experience of nursing in Fair Isle. There are not many young females in the isle and I've been missing out on girlie talk. Edith Ann is a few years younger than me but I'm hoping we can become friends over the holidays.

Once the tables are cleared, it's time for fun and games with the children. Everyone joins in and *The Grand Old Duke of York* and *The Farmer's in the Dell* are firm favourites. The night wears on. And then … it's time for Santie Klaas.

Dodie certainly makes a good one. He's a rotund, jolly man, well-suited to the red suit and false beard. The little children are impressed when he calls them by name and presents them with a surprise gift. Some are brimming with confidence and nearly knock Santie off his feet, while others bury their faces in their mums' bosoms. I love observing the reactions of children. No two are the same. I find it fascinating.

By 8.00pm the little ones are getting tired but are still too excited to want to go home. The band strikes up, and then it's a free-for-all, as the young, the old, toddlers and grandparents all join in the fun. I haven't enjoyed myself like this on a dance floor for a very long time. The Hammersmith Odeon and Chelsea Town Hall, along with the twist, the shake and the jive all pale into insignificance as I reel and jig and let down my hair to the beat of the Fair Isle dance band. There's nothing quite like a good old eightsome reel to get rid of the stress of the last few weeks.

Half-past-eleven on the dot and the frolicking comes to an end. All agree it's been a great night. Tomorrow is Sunday, so the clearing will wait until later in the week. On our way back, mam and dad tell me they have had a great holiday and hope to go back home on Tuesday's *Good Shepherd*. 'We met Tommy's folks at last,' says dad, 'and they've invited us over to Busta tomorrow for a visit.'

The fine weather is holding and there is hardly a breath of wind. I've attended to Jean and finished my routine visits. The sounds of human voices, birds screaming and dogs barking are as clear as bells. I can hear laughter long before I reach Busta.

I enjoy my visits to Busta. It's a bit off the beaten track and, by the time I get there, I'm usually hungry. It's probably the thought of Ellen's home cooking that makes my mouth water. As usual, delicious smells greet me at the door.

'After all, it's Boxing Day,' says Ellen, as she spreads the table with

73

Christmas dinner leftovers. 'We might as well have another party while you folks are here.'

Mam laughs and says that she's done nothing but eat since she arrived in Fair Isle and, if this is what isolation is about, then she's all for it. Dad and Jerry, Tommy's father, are deep in conversation about crofting and fishing. Mam is enjoying looking through Ellen's collection of expertly hand-knitted all-over Fair Isle garments. Ellen tells us how she hand-dyes some of the wool with the extracts of indigenous flowers and plants.

Ellen then suggests that because it's such a fine day we could go for a walk over to Taft, where her brother Sandy and sister Maggie live.

'I would love that,' says mam. 'It'll shake doon some of this food, I hope.'

Dad and Jerry decide to stay behind. I'm sure they're far too comfortable to move.

'Taft is quite a famous house,' says Ellen. 'The royal family visited there in 1960.'

On our way, Ellen tells us about the tragic way Sandy lost his wife Alice and the baby in childbirth. 'He's never got over it, it was terrible. I stayed with her throughout. In fact, I've never got over it myself.'

Ellen is a small, strong, wiry woman, full of beans. Life has certainly had its challenges for her and Jerry. They lost their first-born son, also named Jerry, at the age of 16. 'He died from septicaemia, and just to think it started off with something so simple – a cut finger. It was very hard for wiz, and so sad for Tommy, losing his older brother and best friend.'

Ellen doesn't stay down for long, though. By the time we get to Taft she's back joking and laughing and telling stories about the royal visit. 'The Queen and Prince Phillip wanted to visit a traditional Fair Isle house. Look there, you can see the slate roof and the white-washed walls. It was August 1960, wind was fae da north so the Royal Yacht

Britannia could not come in at North Haven. It was South Harbour or nothing. I'll let Maggie tell you about the visit.'

I've been to Taft many times and I love the atmosphere of the open fire and the crook and I'm now looking forward to showing it off to mam.

CHAPTER 19

As we enter the Taft house, we walk straight back into the 19th century. This classic Fair Isle cottage has been in the Stout family for generations and has been left just as it was built. Within its cosy walls, it's easy to visualise women moving about its kitchen wearing long Victorian dresses, their heads covered by hand-knitted Shetland woollen haps. The men would have been whittling driftwood, making chairs and dressers.

The image fades, but the pot hanging on the crook above the open peat fire is evidence of a bygone era.

Sandy is already at the front door. 'I saw you coming ower. I'm dat blyde you're here.' Sandy and I have a special bond. I see him professionally on a weekly basis. At other times we meet on my rounds, when we stop for a chat. Inevitably, his eyes fill as he recounts over and over again the ordeal of losing his Alice and the baby.

Maggie, Sandy's sister, gives us a warm welcome. 'This is unexpected, you've made wir day. Come in by and have a seat. I'll get tea on the go while we all have a good yarn.'

I can see by the expression on mam's face that she's delighted with

Taft. It's starting to get dark and the Tilley is already lit. Mam says, 'The hiss of the Tilley lamp and the smell of the peat-reek reminds me dat much of my ain childhood home.'

Sandy points out each chair, taking pains to tell us who made it and the year it was made. 'It's all very old fashioned, but we widna give up wir auld hame for a palace.'

'Speaking aboot palaces,' says Ellen, 'Maggie, du'll need to tell Mary aboot the royal visit to this very house.'

'Ach, Ellen, du's far better at the telling than what I am. Du tell, and I'll fill in whit du forgets. After all, it wiz dee that organised all the ladies to bring the homebakes and serve the tea. Dy best china cups and silver teaspoons wir truly fit for a queen.'

Maggie's eyes are twinkling. 'I mind I was brawly nervous, so I wiz ower blyde du wiz here to support me.'

No sooner has Maggie said the words than there's a light knock at the door and Jerry, skipper of the *Good Shepherd*, arrives. Sandy greets his brother and introduces him to mam. 'We were just starting to tell Nurse Mona's mam about the royal visit, so du can add to the story, Jerry.'

Jerry gives a hearty laugh. 'This story has been told many a time.' He goes on to relate how he and Sandy were given the task of transporting the royal family from the South Harbour to Taft. It was decided that Jerry's lorry would do the job. 'Never forget, Sandy, that it was you and me that painted up my old lorry for the royal guests.' A special seat was made by the clerk of works of the National Trust. 'But it wiz me and dee, Sandy, that fitted it on the back of the lorry for the occasion. They seemed pleased enough with our efforts.

'The Royal Yacht *Britannia*, heading south from Lerwick, anchored off the South Harbour. It should have been North Haven, a much bonnier location, but because of the weather that was out of the question and South Harbour it was, on the evening of 11th August 1960.

A party, including the Queen, Prince Phillip, Princess Alexandra and Prince Michael, came ashore by launch. And we greeted them with our shotguns.'

Seeing the look of surprise on our faces, Jerry roars with laughter again. 'No, dunna you worry, we had no intention of killing them. We used our shotguns to give a hearty 21-gun salute.'

Mam is intrigued by the story. 'I can't imagine what you must have been feeling, Ellen. It's not every day you get the chance of entertaining, not only the Queen, but three more close members of the royal family.'

'Well, I got the job of leading the way.' Ellen is smiling hugely at the memory. 'First of all, the Queen requested a visit to an authentic Shetland hoose and Taft, of course, was ideal.'

'I can see that,' says mam. 'The open peat fire, the rafters, the Tilley lamp, and every stick of furniture in here being handmade, you couldn't have chosen better. Keep goin', Ellen, I want to hear more.'

Ellen is happy to explain how she was advised on what the preferences were when it came to the menu, and then again what they couldn't eat, and how the Fair Isle women gave her every support. 'We needn't have worried, because when tea time came they thanked us and, from what they did eat and drink, they seemed to have simple, homely tastes.'

Maggie joins in. 'Oh, she really wiz an afil fine wife, wiz da Queen. Does du ken, Mary, she got doon on her hookers and warmed her hands at my fire? I couldn't believe it. Princess Alexandra, she wiz just lovely too. She asked me all kinds of questions aboot the Fair Isle maakin, and took a big interest in my maakin belt. The twa royal men, well dey wandered aboot da hoose admiring the driftwood furniture and asking questions. When I got a bit flustered, Ellen took over.'

'Maggie, I was proud o dee,' says Ellen. 'Du held dy own. I wiz ower blyde to fill in now and again.'

Sandy joins in, describing the way the isle folk got together to make the hall bonnie, and then the women brought their wires and maakin belts out and put on a demonstration. The royals very kindly and appreciatively accepted knitwear that had been made especially for them.

Jerry laughs. 'Then it was time to get them back on the lorry for their voyage south. Me and you, Sandy, had to hurry back so that we could get to the top of Ward Hill where we, along with lots of folk, lit a celebratory beacon as the *Britannia* departed.'

It's obvious that Ellen has something more on her mind and I guess what's coming next, because I've heard it before. 'Du's no heard the end of it, Mary. Maggie, tell Mary about dee meeting the Queen Mother.' Maggie shakes her head and smiles broadly. It's obvious she's told the tale many a time and I never tire of hearing it.

Two years after the famous visit, Maggie broke her leg. The wind that day was near hurricane-force, which was the reason Maggie fell. She is a petite woman and, as she left the house to fetch a pail of water, the wind blew her over. There was no chance of the *Good Shepherd* attempting a crossing to Grutness. The lifeboat had to be called from Lerwick. Maggie stayed for two months in the Gilbert Bain Hospital while her fracture healed.

'Maggie, du is some woman, drama seems to follow dee around,' says mam.

'Unbeknown to me,' says Maggie, 'the Queen Mother was in Shetland on another royal visit. She came to the ward where I was recuperating and stopped by my bed, and she shook my hand. I'll never forget the look on her face when I told her I had given her daughter tea in my house. I think she thought I wiz doitin. The ward sister put her right, and we all, dat's including the Queen Mother, had a good laugh.'

I check the time and say, 'You'll all be going to the kirk. I'll make my way to Auntie Jean. It's been a great visit, thank you for your kindness. Mam, I'll see you and dad in the morning.'

It's a beautiful, clear, starry night and as I ponder on the Christmas celebrations and the visit to Taft I feel happy and contented.

CHAPTER 20

Monday 27th December. I've been avoiding the thought of mam and dad going back home to Whiteness. I'm going to miss them. I take a deep breath and swallow. No way am I going to allow that familiar lump to rise in my throat. Tomorrow is the big goodbye day and I'm determined to make their last day a happy one.

The fine crisp weather is holding on so once I've had a peerie sleep the three of us, mam, dad and me, go for yet another walk.

'Who would have thought,' says mam, 'on an island as peerie as this, there would be so much to see. The scenery and the cliffs are truly spectacular. You've looked after wiz well, Mona, but now you must be very tired. I'm going back to get wir dinner ready. It's lamb chops again, I'm afraid, but I ken it's your favourite.'

'It's getting better, and there's light at the end of the tunnel as far as Auntie Jean is concerned. I can't leave her during the night because of toileting, though. She's as light as a feather and it's no problem for me to lift her on and off the commode, but I feel it's a bit much for Bab. She is also an auld wife and needs her sleep.'

'Well, as lang as you don't run yourself ragged,' says dad. 'Mind now, you'll be no use to anybody if you get sick.'

'I'll be just fine, don't you worry about me. Mam, if you don't mind, I would like to show dad Stroms Heelor. That's where the Spanish galleon, *El Gran Grifon*, ran aground in 1588. Remember? She was flagship of the Spanish Armada.'

'Off the two of you go, but mind and be home for your dinner.'

Dad and I stroll along, chatting. Dad is pointing out the seabirds screaming and circling above our heads. 'See, Mona, there's the fulmars and the guillemots, and hundreds of gulls joining in the seabird chorus.'

We reach the cliff above Stroms Heelor and, as we peer down to the boiling sea thundering below, dad remarks, 'Between the birds and the sea, this is some noise, is it not?'

We both fall silent. I'm thinking about the sailors on *El Gran Griffon* so many years ago. 'They must have been terrified,' says dad, 'and, of course, what it must have meant for the brave Fair Islanders who risked their lives to rescue them.'

'There's many a story about this incident,' I say. 'Much of it is true, I think, like how the locals took them into their homes until they could be repatriated back to Spain. Then there's the folklore and myths about the women copying the patterns from the flamboyant clothes the Spanish sailors wore, and that was supposedly the basis for Fair Isle maakin'.

Dad laughs, 'Oh, folk will think up many a story for a drama. What du's telling me is far-fetched, I would say. The believable, factual bits are very interesting. But tell me, Mona, I've never had much chance or time for a good old heart-to-heart. How are you really doing?'

'Well, Dad, it's been a bit of a rollercoaster. Some days good, some days bad and some days exciting, especially when I have to draw on my nursing knowledge and come up with an answer. Then again, there are days when I could have killed you stone dead for getting me into this.'

I keep my face deadpan. I watch my father's face pale, his eyes widen and his jaw drop. 'Oh no, no ... ' my dad starts to respond.

I can keep the laughter in no longer, and in no time at all we are both laughing our heads off.

'Oh, du is a bad lass, du is,' dad splutters.

'I think I'm okay, Dad.' I'm serious now, 'For me it's been a maturing process. Professionally, I would never have dreamt of going down this path or, should I say, crossing this sea.'

Dad lifts his eyebrows and gives a smile.

'What would I have done? I really don't know. Probably I would've ended up back in London. Midwifery is my great love, as you know. But here I am, thanks to you.'

'What I've observed, from keeping my eyes and ears open, is that my peerie lass is growing up.'

I gasp as a rush of affection for my dear dad bubbles up from deep inside.

He goes on, 'Many a day I chided myself on insisting you go to Fair Isle. Now, all things considered, I think I was right.'

Dad has a protective arm around me and I'm savouring this conversation. It's a precious time. As we amble along, the thought strikes me that life does have a strange way of dealing out challenges and options. Over the years, dad certainly has dished out a few of these for me. I'm grateful for his guidance.

Tuesday morning. The sky is clear and, oh good, there's not much wind. It's 5.30 and already I have Auntie Jean washed and dressed. Her recovery is slow but steady and we can converse. 'Mam and dad are going back to Shetland today,' I tell her, as I spoon milky porridge into her eager mouth. I'm pleased that her appetite is improving.

'You'll miss them, I'm sure,' Auntie Jean's words come out breathy and slow. 'I did enjoy their visits. Give them my love.'

'I will do that, Auntie Jean. I'm going now to see them off. I'll call

Bab, mind and have a peerie sleep. I'll come along on my way home.'

'I think you're going to hae a fine trip in,' says young Stewart as he stows mam and dad's luggage safely into the back of his pick-up.

'I hope so, Stewart,' I can see a look of relief on mam's face. I know she is dreading a stormy journey for dad. Mam has never experienced seasickness in her life. I know who I inherited my battle with seasickness from.

We keep the goodbyes short. 'It'll not be too long before your holidays are due,' says mam, kissing my cheek.

'Stewart, it's a bonnie day, I'll walk back home. The fresh air will do me good.' I give dad a hug and say a quick 'cheerio' to both my folks. Halfway along the jetty I can't resist another look back. They're already on the deck of the *Good Shepherd* and standing close, dad with his arm around mam. I can't see mam's tears but I know they're there. I can feel them on my own cheeks.

CHAPTER 21

During January, gales in Shetland are legendary, reaching storm- and sometimes hurricane-force. I've spent so many years away from Shetland I've all but forgotten just how ferocious wind speeds can be. Here in Fair Isle there is no getting away from it and, in a quirky way, I'm enjoying braving the elements.

My friends, the two Stewarts, go out of their way to accommodate me when I need a lift. If my patient lives in an awkward location, where no vehicle can reach and the wind speed is high, they are on hand to help. As young Stewart puts it, 'I'm here to give dee something to haad on tae.'

As I hoped, while she's on school holidays Edith Ann is my companion. She brightens my days and I have a warm feeling that I've made a friend for life. I repeatedly tell her she would make an ideal nurse. 'I'll give it some thought,' she says, cautiously, with a twinkle in her eye.

Today it's Edith Ann's dad, Jimmy, who knocks loudly on my door. I abandon my lunch. There is urgency in that knock and something is telling me that trouble is brewing.

'It's Sandy,' says Jimmy, without preamble. 'I happened to go by Taft just a peerie start ago. Sandy is not well, his head is splitting and he feels very hot to my touch, so I told him to lie down and I'd go and fetch dee.'

Jimmy hurries along with me to Taft. 'Sandy, I've brought Nurse Mona. I'll leave you now, but if you need any assistance, Mona will lat me ken.'

Sandy nods but doesn't answer. Maggie is visibly upset. 'He didn't have a good night, and he kept calling for me to sit with him. This morning he was no better. I was dat relieved when Jimmy cam by.'

'Well, Maggie, I'll see what I can do for Sandy, and dan we'll tak it fae dere.' I say this with confidence, as much to reassure myself as her. Inside, I'm not so sure about the situation.

'I'm blyde you're here, Nurse. I can relax now.'

I take a couple of minutes to comfort Maggie. 'You sit by the fire and once I've examined Sandy I'll join you and lat you ken what I think.'

The first thing I note as I approach Sandy's bed is his dislike of light. He screws up his eyes and turns his head away from the daylight streaming in the window. This could well be a clue to what is wrong with Sandy. As soon as the thought crosses my mind, I dismiss it. Take your time, Mona, I tell myself severely. No jumping to diagnostic conclusions. Go easy and think logically before you call Dr Mainland.

Sandy is ill, there's no doubt about it. 'Sandy, I'm sorry du's feeling so miserable. I'll need to examine dee afore I report back to Dr Mainland. First of all, I'll need to take your temperature and feel your pulse.'

Sandy is reluctant to open his mouth. In fact, he seems a bit confused. I change my mind and slip the thermometer under his armpit. His pulse is rapid and his hands and feet are cold. The thermometer reads 101.2F.

'Could you try a drink of water, Sandy?' He nods a yes. 'Very good then, I can see you're thirsty.' He's also dehydrated. Unfortunately, when I encourage him to drink he can't swallow for retching. My heart sinks as he pushes my hand away.

I call Maggie into the bedroom and give them my opinion. I hold Sandy's hand and say, 'Sandy, I think you'll have to go to hospital. I'll check this with Dr Mainland and I'm sure he'll agree that the best place for you is the Gilbert Bain.'

'All right, Nurse.' Sandy squeezes my hand. 'You do what you think is right.' His voice is now a mere whisper.

I must get a move on. I remember listening to the weather forecast this morning and hearing, 'Fair Isle, wind freshening to force 5 to 6.' I'm hoping the *Good Shepherd* will make the trip. If not, there is always the lifeboat from Lerwick, but that will take time and, in this case, I'm thinking time is of the essence.

'It doesn't sound good, Nurse Smith,' says Dr Mainland. 'You say his neck is stiff, and he doesn't like the light?'

'Yes, Doctor, he also seems confused and he's nauseous. I'm worried about hydration. From my observations, it would appear that perhaps it's meningitis?' There, I've said it.

'And with that high temperature there could be a danger of septi-caemia. It certainly does sound like it could well be meningitis. Phone back once you've confirmed that the *Good Shepherd* can go. If so, I'll arrange an ambulance to meet you at Grutness and I'll book a bed for Sandy at the Gilbert Bain.'

'Thanks, Dr Mainland. I'll get things going as quick as I can and will get back to you.'

I go to Midway and tell Jimmy the news.

'I've been expecting this. I'm skipper on call, so I'll round up the crew and we'll be on wir way. Thank goodness the wind is not too bad. A bit much for you, Nurse Mona, but I know you'll come with us. As long as you can look after Sandy, we'll look after you.'

'Thanks, Jimmy. I'll get Sandy ready. He's not fit enough to stand or walk and he'll need a stretcher. I'll phone Dr Mainland and tell him we're going. I'll ask Stewart to take the stretcher in his lorry to Taft. Young Stewart will give a hand, I'm sure. You and the crew will be busy getting the *Good Shepherd* ready for the trip.'

Back at Taft I break the news. Maggie is relieved and Sandy seems resigned. I tell him I'm going to give him a strong pain-killing injection along with one to combat his nausea. I detect a smile as he nods his head and squeezes my hand.

I don't have time to worry about the sea and Da Roost. I know the crew will have to get Sandy and the stretcher down into the hold and that's going to take skill and know-how. I'll take blankets and buckets for both Sandy and me, and I'll try my best to keep a semblance of dignity. I laugh out loud at my thoughts.

I make myself a bed alongside Sandy's stretcher. The injections have taken effect and Sandy is fast asleep. I'm thankful for small mercies. Being a Fair Isle man, Sandy is not prone to seasickness. It's a blessing as he has more than enough to cope with.

I listen to the sound of chains and many more unidentifiable noises far above me. I hear the crew talking and someone shouting orders. The engine starts and ... oh no, I forgot about the diesel. The smell is overpowering. Oh well, in for a penny, in for a pound.

It's not a good trip. The sea is very rough and I am very sick. Fortunately, I don't have to do very much for Sandy. His loud snoring is all I need to tell me he's breathing. I'm ashamed to acknowledge that I'm feeling very sorry for myself as I cling tightly onto the old National Dried Milk tin. This is by far my worst *Good Shepherd* trip yet. She's bucking and rolling and I'm convinced she's standing on her head. Any minute now, I'm thinking, she's going to the bottom of the sea. In fact, I wish she would sink and put me out of my misery.

I open my eyes and look over at Sandy. He's calm and peaceful, with a beatific smile pulling on the corners of his mouth. It's the morphine, I'm sure. Wish I had given myself one before I left the isle. Ha, I'm going a bit crazy. Then we hit Da Roost and that's another story.

I see a pair of legs descending the ladder, and there's my knight in shining oilskins. 'Oh, Tommy, have we got far to go?' It's a childish question, I know, but I'm beyond caring.

'Is du aright?' Tommy's strong features soften, and I can see he's feeling sorry for me. 'Daft question. I can see du's feeling like death. It's not long now and we'll be at the Grutness pier. Du's doing just fine. Hang in dere.'

And with that, Tommy is up the ladder again, leaving me with an over-abundance of self-pity.

Oh, thank goodness, Grutness at last. I hear banging and shouting and chains rattling. The next problem for me is to get myself onto my feet. I pull my knees up, roll over and deliberately haul myself up to my feet. I hang on tight to the rail and test my balance. My legs are shaky, so I do a bit of gentle running. No, not running, more like stumbling on the spot.

Tommy is back in the hold. 'I'll give dee a hand up to the top deck, wait up there, and mind and take some good refreshing breaths. As soon as we can, we'll have Sandy up beside dee.'

Sure enough, the ambulance is waiting and in no time at all Sandy is safe and sound. To say I'm relieved is an understatement. As I hand over my observation report to the ambulance driver, I ask him to give me five minutes with Sandy before he drives off.

'Well, Nurse, your patient looks fine. I can't say the same about you, though.' He smiles cheekily at me. 'Maybe you should come along with me to the hospital for admission?'

I take a swipe at him and give a feeble smile. 'You're a cheeky one, you are, for sure. Hold fire till I say goodbye to my patient.'

Sandy is awake and lucid. His voice is still weak and there are those familiar tears welling up in his eyes. 'Thank you so much, mind and be in the isle to greet me when I come hame.'

'Of course I will, Sandy.' And throwing all professional caution to the wind, I kiss the top of his sore head.

CHAPTER 22

The fearsome January gales have given way to a snowy and icy February. It's much better for my temperament, as the wind unsettles me. Three times during January the *Good Shepherd* was held up. Twice she made the trip after a few days, but on one occasion the isle was cut off for over a week.

That week tested my nerves and my confidence. I listened obsessively to the weather forecast, hoping the wind would ease. No such luck. The weather gods were not listening, so I sat it out and prayed to my God. I would wake up during the night, sometimes in a cold sweat. Blood, heart attacks and broken bones haunted my dreams. I constantly had to remind myself that these were just fantasies, and this was exhausting in itself.

Sheila is 36 weeks pregnant now. It's time for her to leave the isle to have her baby. I have become very fond of Sheila and Stewart Wilson. I hope my antenatal care and childbirth education will help her through when the time comes. We've had lots of fun over the past seven months. I'll miss her.

'I'm feeling a bit nervous,' she tells me, 'but you've prepared me well. I'll miss Stewart like mad. It's unfortunate he can't come with me, but he has to mind the shop.'

'It's such a pity. I'm sorry, but as you say, needs must.'

But, at last the weather has settled and I'm enjoying sledging. Stewart is accompanying me on my rounds. We fill up Stewart's sledge with necessities from the shop – milk, bread, tea and so on – and off we go from house to house, making sure their occupants' needs, both physical and medical, are being met. Once the sledge is empty, I take my place on it and Stewart pulls me along just for fun.

'I'm missing Sheila,' Stewart confides, and I know he's feeling a bit lost without his wife. 'Pulling you along on my sledge takes my mind off worrying about her.'

'I'm sure she'll be fine, Stewart. Just think about your brand-new baby. We'll need to have a party once they're back.'

Auntie Jean has rallied. She's still top priority on my nursing care list, though. Bab never fails to amaze me and has insisted that her bed be brought into the ben room so she can attend Jean during the night. It's good to see Bab animated. She's confined to the house, and I'm concerned that she might be feeling a bit down. I needn't have worried. 'I'm enjoying looking after Jean,' she tells me. 'I always wanted to be a nurse, and now I've got the chance.'

After much care and persuasion, Bab and I have finally got Jean up and out of bed. 'You're doing just fine, Auntie Jean,' I say over and over. 'Take care and mind your step, Bab and me are right here, we'll no let you faa.' Bab now manages to do this without my help.

'Guid bless you, I never did think I would ever be up again.' Auntie Jean loves sitting by the fire for short spells. Her voice is stronger, her appetite continues to improve, and I'm happy she's on the mend.

As if the snow isn't enough to contend with, the dreaded flu strikes the isle. Leogh Willie wasn't far wrong. I've had flu once or twice during my life, but generally I'm fit and healthy, so I'm hoping I don't succumb. An ill nurse isn't much use to anyone. I'm concentrating on keeping my immune system in good order. A healthy diet, exercise and sleep are high on my agenda.

It's a busy time. The Fair Isle folk are considerate and, rather than call in their busy nurse, many treat themselves with rest and aspirin and after a few days are back on their feet. However, some are so ill and miserable they need house visits. My two peerie Viking boys, Michael and Kenneth, both go down with whooping cough. They are strong wee guys and warmth, bed rest, plenty of fluids and Linctus Codeine every four hours, prescribed by Dr Mainland, soon sees them right. My concern is for the very young and the elderly.

Again, Stewart comes to the rescue, accompanying me on my daily rounds, making sure fires are lit, animals are fed and cupboards stocked, if that's what's needed. I visit Leogh Willie and remind him of how he challenged me with the milking of cows and feeding of hens.

'Naa, naa, Nurse ... ' He laughs heartily, 'I'm doing ower weel, bidin in me bed. I have nae animals to worry about, but I'm ower blyde Stewart can see to me fire.'

My big fear, of course, is Auntie Jean. If she gets the flu in her condition it will surely kill her. I suggest to Bab and Willum that we isolate Lower Staneybrake. No visitors, just myself and Stewart.

'Whatever you think, Nurse. Me and Bab will go along with your advice.' Willum gives a smile, 'But it's all this washing of hands. We're not going to have a flake of skin left on them.'

CHAPTER 23

February is flying past. Because I'm busy, I seldom have time to note what day, let alone what date it is. The snow has disappeared but it's very cold and icy. While walking the fields and the road, I constantly remind myself to be careful. The *Good Shepherd* is on schedule. Tuesday and Friday are her days, and she manages somehow to scrape together a crew, despite the flu taking its toll.

I love the bright blue sky above and the crackling frost beneath my feet. In an unofficial capacity, I often pop in on the elderly, vulnerable folk. I've been to Helen and Lottie today, making sure their health is good and that they're coping.

'Thank you for minding on wiz,' said Helen. 'We're fine, really we are, keeping snug by the fire till this flu taks aff. We're dat thankful we've no caught it.'

'Thankful we've no caught it,' repeated Lottie.

I've finished my dinner and I'm curled up in my comfy chair by the Rayburn, sipping hot cocoa. It's been a busy time and I'm tired. The phone rings. It's Jack McPherson, lighthouse keeper.

'Sorry to bother you, Nurse, but Margaret is not feeling well. This flu doesn't want to lift, and her chest is sore.'

'No bother at all, Jack. I'll be beside you as soon as I can.' I pull on a warm track suit, get my medical bag ready and prepare for the trudge to the South Lighthouse. Before I set off, though, I call on Annie to tell her where I'm going.

'Stewart can give you a lift,' she says.

'No, Annie I'll be fine, and in any case the road will be icy. I don't want the pick-up to slide. I've got my torch and I'll be careful.'

I am careful, although I walk as fast as I can. It's a beautiful, still night, the moon is waning and I'm sorely tempted to lift my eyes to the heavens, but common sense prevails and I keep them firmly on my heavy boots, in case I slip.

Margaret McPherson is nearly eight months pregnant and is preparing to leave Fair Isle to go south to her parents. I've booked her into a maternity hospital in her home town. Now this illness might complicate matters.

When I arrive at the McPhersons', Jack is clearing up in the kitchen. He gives me a warm welcome. Wee lass Millie knows me well. She is going south with her mum, to be looked after by her granny while Margaret has the baby. I spend a few minutes chatting and joking with Millie before turning my attention to Margaret.

'We were so thankful none of us got the flu. Then Margaret went down with it.' It's obvious that Jack is more than a little worried. I suggest he stays with Millie until I've done my observations.

'Let me take a look at Margaret, Jack. Then we'll take it from there.'

The bedroom is hot and stuffy. I can see immediately that Margaret isn't well. She's flushed and fevered and has a harsh cough.

'As I say, Margaret, you've really done well during your pregnancy. I'm so sorry you're now feeling poorly. I'll examine you, and then I'll let you know what I come up with.'

I pop the thermometer under her tongue and, while it's registering,

I gently poke and prod her tummy and listen in to the baby's heartbeat. 'All fine down this end but, oh dear, your temperature is over 100. I'll get you a glass of water and give you a quick sponge down.'

'Thank you. That sounds heavenly,' she says. 'I'm feeling hot and sticky. Please would you open the window? Jack has a thing about me catching cold.'

I call Jack, who duly opens the window and tenderly helps Margaret to drink a full glass of water. I take time to sponge Margaret and change her nightie, while murmuring words of encouragement. I look in Margaret's ears, eyes and throat, and listen in to her chest. I breathe a sigh of relief. I was dreading a chest infection. But thank goodness, her chest sounds are clear.

Expressions of anxiety and expectation flit across Margaret's face. I sit down on her bed, take her hot hand in mine, and give my verdict to both her and Jack.

'I do think it's just a nasty dose of flu. Your chest is clear. That's the good news.'

'Is there bad news, then?' Both Jack and Margaret say in unison.

I go on to explain that any infection is not good news during pregnancy. 'There's the risk of premature labour. I'll discuss this with Dr Mainland. I'm sure he'll agree to put you on antibiotics, Margaret. Flu is caused by a virus, so antibiotics are not helpful. But in your case, he'll maybe prescribe them as prevention against secondary infection.'

Tears well up in Margaret's eyes, and I think they're not far from Jack's either.

When we finish up, Jack tells me he'd like to accompany me home. 'The roads are icy and I want to be of help.'

'I'll take you up on that, Jack. We'll get going and, Margaret, we'll be back as soon as we can.'

Jack goes next door and has a word with Mrs Smith, a kindly neighbour, who is more than willing to keep an eye on Margaret and Millie.

I've got to know Jack McPherson well. Since Margaret confided in me about her postnatal depression, I've made a point of discussing this condition with both her and Jack. They are aware, and understand, that the condition may not affect Margaret this time, but if it does, they will be open about it and seek help.

Jack and I discuss this subject while we trundle back to my house. It's slow going, but it gives us time to have an in-depth conversation.

'I hope and pray all will go well,' Jack says. I can see he's doing his best to keep his fears at bay. I can think of nothing to say to reassure him.

'Oh, it's you, Nurse,' Dr Mainland seems a bit surprised. It's 9.30pm and I'm guessing he's settled down, contemplating a quiet night with his family. Then here I come, disturbing the peace. I quickly fill him in on the details of Margaret's condition.

'Yes. Yes, I agree,' he says. 'She's 36 weeks, what we don't want is a premature baby in Fair Isle. And you're right about the antibiotics. We certainly don't want Margaret developing a secondary infection.'

'I'll get going with the antibiotics then. I'll keep an eagle eye on her, and hopefully she'll be well enough for the trip on the *Good Shepherd* on Friday.'

As I prepare the medications and get ready for the walk back to the South Lighthouse with Jack, a thought occurs to me. The conversation with Dr Mainland has boosted my confidence. I took the lead, and Dr Mainland seemed happy I did. It's a small step in the right direction.

After living for six months in Fair Isle, one of the things I have learnt is to pay attention to my intuition, my gut feeling.

On the way back I get a sense that Jack wants to open up about something. Sure enough, halfway down the road, he stops. He takes a deep breath, lets the air out with a loud sigh, and then it comes out. 'I haven't told a soul, not even Margaret, I don't want to get her hopes up and then have them dashed. I've applied for a transfer.'

I first reassure Jack that this information will stay with me, then stand stock-still in the hope that he'll feel comfortable enough to enlarge on the story.

'I've been a lighthouse keeper since I left school. I'm very happy in my job. The problem is Fair Isle. I love it here, but it's too isolated, and I know Margaret misses her family. It's a hassle getting the family off the isle, then on to the 'north boat' and down to Aberdeen. If my application is successful I'm hoping to get a post on the Scottish mainland, and then at least we'll have a better family life.'

I tell Jack that he knows what's best. 'Meantime, we'll get Margaret settled and, hopefully, on her way to recovery.'

My visit to the lighthouse on Thursday afternoon means I have to make the decision on whether Margaret is fit enough for the long journey tomorrow. It turns out she's getting better, but is not well enough to travel. Jack now has the flu and Millie is sniffling.

'We'll hang on till next Tuesday,' I tell them, reluctantly. 'By which time I'm sure you'll be ready to leave.' I say this with more confidence than I feel. Some things in life are beyond my control, I tell myself. But by Monday, Margaret is much better and Jack is trying hard to make light of his illness. 'Normally, I wouldn't let you go,' I tell them. 'But I think it best you get yourselves settled with your mum, Margaret, and then you'll be in easy reach of the hospital.'

Early Tuesday morning, young Stewart is up and ready to take the McPhersons on the first stage of their journey. Margaret and Millie squeeze in the front beside Stewart, while Jack and I huddle in the back. Stewart drives along very slowly and very carefully. 'I have precious cargo aboard this morning,' he says, with a smile.

I make sure Margaret is warm and comfortable in the lower bunk on the *Good Shepherd*, with Millie cuddled in beside her. Jack takes his place on the upper bunk. I can see he's happy to get his head down. His flu is all too evident.

While the crew are getting the vessel ready to disembark, I take time to have a word with Margaret. 'You have my letter for the midwife who will be looking after you. In it, I've told her about your previous postnatal depression. Dr Mainland can be contacted by the hospital if they need any more information.'

'Thank you, Mona.' Margaret is tearful and tells me she has appreciated my care and will never again hold back. She will express exactly how she feels.

'Good for you,' I reply. 'I'm here for you, if you have any concerns give me a ring, day or night.'

I don't mention seasickness but say a silent prayer that they're spared. I say goodbye, reminding myself again that some things are out of my control.

CHAPTER 24

.

February is drawing to a close and the days are lengthening ever so slightly. I'm not a fan of winter, so now that spring is on the way I'm feeling happier. Fortunately, the frosty weather is still holding on and that keeps the wind at bay.

I'm having a bit of a respite. I've 'lost' my two pregnant mums, Auntie Jean is stronger, and the flu has all but disappeared, so I've little to worry about.

I love the clear, starry nights. It's one of the perks of winter. On these quiet evenings I take my binoculars and head to various spots on the isle, just to look up and wonder at the world above.

I keep hoping I'm going to see the northern lights or, should I say, the mirrie dancers as they're called in Shetland. Magnificent celestial beings that they are, I'm fascinated by them. But they are notoriously difficult to predict. They love playing tricks and hide away just when you think they're going to show off. I keep hoping, though.

Tonight I pop in to say hello to Auntie Jean, Bab and Willum. I've lifted the isolation ban.

'I'm really blyde that the flu has taen aff, and that it never came wir wye.' Willum gives me a huge smile and a wink.

'Oh, yes, indeed, Willum. So am I.' I let out a sigh of relief that's not lost on Auntie Bab. I wish them goodnight and make my way southward to my house.

For some inexplicable reason, I turn around and ... and, oh boy! The north sky is ablaze with every colour imaginable, dancing and flitting across the sky. Red and green streamers leave the heavens and swirl their way to earth. The well-named mirrie dancers at last, tripping the light fantastic. I feel as if they are putting on a show just for me. I stand in awe. Oh, how I wish dad were here beside me to enjoy this spectacle.

Time is marching on. I have but three months left of my Fair Isle contract. What do I want to do once the time is up? The truth is that I've no idea. I tuck the question away in the back of my mind. I'll think about it nearer the time. Meantime, I'm going through a quiet spell and enjoying it. The month of March officially heralds spring, not that I'd know it from the constant rain and never-ending wind.

Good news comes my way on 19th March, and it cheers me up no end. Stewart Wilson bursts into my kitchen to tell me – 'I just couldn't wait ... it's a boy!'

'Oh, Stewart, that's the best news I've heard for ages.' Then the two of us are laughing with joy. 'Are they both well?'

'Yes, they are. I'm thrilled to bits. I knew you would want to hear the news straight away.'

CHAPTER 25

Just when I think I've got it all together, and my life stable and ordered, I'm in for an unexpected shock.

It's a gusty day, perfect for getting my washing dry. I'm busy hanging my clothes on the line when I see Auntie Bab coming my way. She's trying hard to hurry, but age is catching up with her. I know immediately something is amiss. I drop the wash basket and sprint to meet her. Bab is shaking, her face is flushed and she's very agitated.

'Now, Bab, come in and have a seat and tell me what's wrong.'

Gently, I usher Bab into the clinic room. In between the sobbing I piece together what the problem is.

'It's Jean.'

'Okay, Bab, what's happened?'

'I got her up at about half-past-five this morning, as usual. She seemed fine and we even had a peerie conversation.'

Bab blows her nose and hiccoughs. I put my arm around her shoulder. 'Take your time, and when you're ready, tell me more.' I'm trying my best to keep steady, but at the same time I desperately need to know what's wrong.

'Well, I got her back in the bed. Sometimes she'll sleep for a good four hours before she wakes again, so I thought nothing of it. By ten-past-ten I went to see how she was, and then, and then ... '

'You're doing fine, Bab. What happened after that?'

'I couldn't rouse her at all. I couldn't wake her up so I ran to get Willum. He's with her now, and he told me to go and get you. I was dat blyde when I saw you out at da claes line.'

Leaving Bab, I run next door. Sure enough, Annie is busy in the post office, and for once there are no customers. I quickly tell Annie the story and ask her to please keep an eye on Bab as I'll need to get to Lower Staneybrake as fast as I can.

I grab my medical bag and off I go, at the gallop. I spot Willum by the front door and he raises his hand in a wave. He greets me with a pat on the shoulder, his usual smiley face solemn. 'Come you awa ben and take a look at her.'

Jean is lying on her back and breathing heavily. 'Hello, Auntie Jean, it's Nurse Mona here, how are you?'

No response. I can see at once that she's had a stroke. The right side of her face shows the classic droop, and her right arm is limp. I try to get a response but there's nothing. She's unconscious.

I force myself to go through the routine observations. Not much point, but I must do it. Temperature, pulse, blood pressure, reflexes. I record everything accurately. Willum is watching my every move, standing silently by the side of her bed.

I straighten Jean's nightie and bed-clothes, I clean her dentures and moisten her mouth, and make sure she's not in pain. And that's about it. Then I take Willum's hand. 'Come you, we'll take a seat in the kitchen and then I'll make us both a cup of tea.'

Cups of tea must surely be every nurse's back-up plan. I remember a few years back when I had to console a young widow after her husband died. Weeks later she came to see me and presented me with a box of chocolates. 'The one thing, Nurse, that I'll never forget when the doctor came to tell me the bad news, it was that warm cup of tea you brought, along with your kindness. That got me through. I wrapped both my hands around that cup and kept squeezing it for comfort. Thank you so much.'

Willum and I sit by the kitchen fire. I take another peep at Jean, but there's no change, no response. I note that Willum has his hands around his mug of tea.

'Willum, I'm afraid it's no looking good. Jean's had a stroke and I do think it's just a matter of time. Efter aa you've been through I'm so very vexed and sorry.' It's me that is fighting the tears now. 'I'm going to phone Dr Mainland. I'll no be lang, and I'll bring Bab back with me.'

As I stand up, Willum comes over and puts his arm around my shoulder. I notice his strong, gnarled hand; the hand that's made many a coffin. Oh, Willum, Willum, I'm thinking, and then my tears flow.

'Now, Mona, you've done well fur wiz. No need to be sorry. This borrowed time I've had wi my Jean has been a joy. I'm ready now to lat her go.' He smiles at me and squeezes my shoulder.

I pull myself together before lifting the phone to make contact with Dr Mainland. What on earth would he think if I told him that, instead of the nurse comforting the relative, the relative of the patient ends up comforting the nurse? Well, he never need know, and I can bet on it that Uncle Willum will never say a word.

I tentatively wind the phone handle and Annie puts me through. 'Hello, Nurse Smith, what can I do for you today?'

I can tell by the tone of his voice that he's busy, and I remind myself to keep it short and to the point. 'It's not good news, Doctor. It's Jean and, from what I observe, she's had a severe stroke and she's unconscious.'

'Oh, oh, yes, I see. Not good, as you say. Keep all your notes and records in order. Now, Jean herself, what do you think?'

'Well, I think it's just a matter of time. I also think it won't be long, as she hasn't much strength left. She's still recovering from the chest infection and, as you know, she's very frail.'

'By what you're telling me, I do think it's a case of keeping Jean as comfortable as you know how. I'm on the end of this phone if you need my advice.'

After thanking Dr Mainland, I go next door and tell Annie my concerns. I'm feeling a bit shaky and wise Annie's reassurance is what I need. 'We are all here ready and waiting to give Willum and Bab, and you of course, Mona, a hand where needed. Let's just take it day by day.'

Telling Bab the news about her sister is much easier than I anticipated. The problem for Bab is a feeling of guilt. 'Oh, if only I had bidden wi her, and kept my eye on her, I might have been able to call for you sooner.'

'Now, Bab, put that thought right out of your mind. Jean wouldn't have known a thing. Most probably, when the stroke came, she would have been asleep.'

'Oh, I am blyde to hear you say dat. Could I have done anything at all?'

'No, Bab, Jean's time has come. There's nothing that you, or I for that matter, could have done.'

Back in Lower Staneybrake I stay with Jean for a bit. Willum and Bab settle down in the kitchen and, after some time, I join them so that we can work out a plan.

'It's back to where we were the last time Auntie Jean fell ill. Fortunately, da wadder is not as bad as it was then. I'll sit with her all night and then, if you both can be with her during the day, that would be just fine.'

After much debate, both Willum and Bab agree to my suggestion. I tell them I will speak with Tommy and young Stewart and with

Stewart and Annie, and I'm sure they'll agree to call in at certain times during the day to see how things are going.

I put a notice on my front door, the shop and the post office, to let folks know that I am at Lower Staneybrake. Auntie Jean remains critical but stable. I spend the day reassuring and comforting. Willum and Bab look lost so I quickly devise a plan and ask them to sit by Jean's bed.

'The best thing you can do is to hold her hand and speak to her. I really don't know how much she'll be able to hear, but tell her what's on your heart.'

Time passes slowly. Bab once again comes to the fore, helping me with basic nursing care. She yarns away to her sister about times past and, now and again, she gives a chuckle. Once Bab and I have done our bit, we leave Willum with his wife. It's a private, intimate time for them, so we make ourselves scarce.

Sure enough, my helpers are calling in and visiting, finding out how we're doing. Mrs Brown calls along after school has closed. She is the schoolteacher and we have become firm friends. She's an interesting woman, having taught in a school for the blind in Edinburgh before she and her husband, Reverend Brown, the Church of Scotland minister, came to Fair Isle. We spend an hour chatting.

'Are you sure you're up for the night shift, Mona?'

'It really isn't a problem for me. I'm one of these crazy nurses who enjoys night duty, and I have no problem sleeping during the day. Truth to tell, I have no problem sleeping, day or night.'

By 10pm Willum and Bab are tucked up in bed. 'I promise I'll call you if there is any change,' I reassure them.

'Are you sure?' Willum is concerned. 'It would be no trouble for me to sit aa night we Jean.'

'We don't know what tomorrow might bring, so you need to be well rested, both of you. Try and get some sleep if you can.'

Annie has brought me books and magazines and I have my diary to keep me going and awake during the wee small hours. She's also brought my knitting, an attempt at an all-over Fair Isle jumper. 'Oh, Annie, I'm so embarrassed. I didn't want anybody, let alone you, to see my handiwork.'

We both have a good giggle. 'I'll mak a Fair Isle knitter o dee yet, Mona.'

Apart from the rain lashing on the ben window, all is quiet and the night passes. At 6.30am I turn Jean over and massage her pressure points. It's then that her breathing changes. I've heard this breathing pattern many times and I know it's an indication that death is near.

Before calling Willum, I take a few minutes just to be with my dear friend Jean, because that is what I view her to be. Over these past months she has ceased to be simply a patient, and has become a friend.

Although I have attended deathbeds many times, I have never attended a death at home. Hospital deaths are viewed as routine. Often, relatives are not present and we nurses are not encouraged to show emotion. A stiff upper lip is all-important. I've heard and read recently about a woman by the name of Cicely Saunders who is doing research into the care given to the terminally ill. It would seem that the medical and nursing fraternities are falling far short on compassionate care, and symptom control.

Well, it's about time, I'm thinking, that we nurses do show our emotions in a loving, kind way. I realise that I'm going to do just that. I'm privileged to be here in Fair Isle. I have all the time in the world, there is no rush.

I call Willum.

CHAPTER 26

I gently close Auntie Jean's eyes and a thought comes to mind: to be present at the closing of the eyes of the departed and the opening of the eyes of the new-born is a privilege that I will never again take for granted.

I note the time: 11.25 on 29th March 1966.

For the next couple of hours I sit in the kitchen with Bab and Willum while we warm our hands on our mugs of tea. The air is cold despite the warm fire. There's something missing – even the sturdy old table and the driftwood dresser are looking forlorn – of course, it's Jean's presence. Or perhaps we're registering her absence. We talk slowly and quietly.

Willum is relaxed and, giving a tentative smile, he looks me in the eye. 'That's life playing out. A birth and a death in the last ten days: baby Steven Wilson enters our world, and my Jean leaves.'

The three of us become a little philosophical and discuss life and death and what makes it worthwhile. I must say, I always learn something from the old folks and never tire of our conversations. I then ask Bab if she would help me with the last offices for Jean.

'What does du mean by last offices?'

'Sorry, Bab, I'm feeling a bit tired. I should never have used the term. It's a lofty one that we nurses use. It simply means, care of the person who has passed away. It's my duty as the nurse to do this, with reverence and dignity, but it's not a duty for me, it's a privilege.'

Of course, there's more to it. There are the legal issues such as recording the time, the date, the cause of death and the signing of the death certificate, not to mention being properly respectful of religious and cultural beliefs. 'I'll carry on the nursing care, as usual,' I add. 'It would be great if you could help me?'

Bab agrees. 'I'm blyde to be able to do this for Jean. Haad du on, I'll get things ready, little did I ken du wid ask me to help. I'm truly honoured.'

We strip the bed and make it up with brand-new linen. We wash Jean and dress her in a soft, cosy nightie.

'Whit tinks du o dis bonnie een, Mona? Bab holds up a pink lace bed-jacket. It wiz a favourite of hers.'

'It's lovely, Bab.' We gently arrange Jean's arms and tie the silk bows. 'I'm blyde she enjoyed it while she was still with us.'

We comb and braid Jean's hair. Bab has remained stoical and dignified throughout. She smiles. 'I feel better. You've helped me, thank you.' I note a single tear on her cheek. We leave Jean looking peaceful and relaxed.

Funeral rituals differ according to culture. When I was a child in Shetland, women and children didn't participate. The nearest male relative would organise proceedings, including the funeral and interment. Change is on the way now and some women attend the church service but still do not continue to the graveside. Children are kept well clear. The thinking is they should be protected from the sadness.

Never having been to a funeral, I am no expert. The thought suddenly strikes: I should've asked what would be expected of me – if anything – at Jean's funeral. Tommy and his dad Jerry, Jean's brother, will be visiting soon. I decide I'll pick Tommy's brains on the subject before I finally go home and report the death to Dr Mainland.

Tommy's parents, Ellen and Jerry, join Willum and Bab at Jean's bedside. Tommy and I have a heart-to-heart at the kitchen table. 'You've done your bit, Mona, now you can retire for a peerie start.'

Tommy smiles and, restraining his hearty laugh he goes on, 'When it comes to funerals, here in Fair Isle women take a back seat while we men get on with things.' He tells me that today will be a quiet day. Family and friends will visit Lower Staneybrake to offer support and condolences.

Tomorrow, the grave will be dug and the coffin will be made. Depending on their various skills, work will be divided between the able-bodied men. 'Uncle has the wood ready on the laft. If du happens to pass by, du'll probably hear a lot of banging. Once the kist is complete it'll be covered in black cloth, which is tacked on to the wood. Uncle and dad will lay Auntie Jean in, and then the lid will be nailed down.'

I'm happy Jean is cosy in her bonnie nightie. 'Thanks for telling me this, Tommy. I do appreciate it, it's not an easy subject.'

'It's all about practicalities,' Tommy continues. 'Eight of us will carry da kist from here to the kirk, and there Auntie Jean will lie until Saturday, funeral day. Reverend Brown will take the service, both in the kirk and at the graveside. We'll take turns to carry the kist to the cemetery.'

I ponder on what Tommy has told me. The simplicity of the funeral appeals to me. It's then that I make a spontaneous decision. I feel cheated that I can't be there when Auntie Jean is finally laid to rest so I'm going to find a spot where I can look down on the cemetery, I'm sure my trusty binoculars will help in my surreptitious plan. I put this thought aside for the moment as Tommy adds, 'No flowers or wreaths.

After the burial, we'll all go back home and carry on our day as usual. A tombstone will be erected in time.'

I'm exhausted. I say my farewells and make my way home on tired legs to mourn in private.

Dr Mainland listens intently. 'So, she's gone. How are you doing, and how are the report notes looking?'

'I'm fine, Dr Mainland, feeling rather tired. I'm looking forward to a good night's sleep. I've written down all the relevant observations.'

'I'll take it from there,' Dr Mainland says. 'I'll look after the legalities. By the way, we've not met each other. How long is it now since you arrived in Fair Isle?'

Annie's face comes to mind and I remember her saying, 'If he learns to trust you, he'll come less and less.'

'Eight months ... ' I leave the words hanging in the air.

'Is it really that long? I've been intending to come in and meet you and do a round of the patients. Tell you what, I have plans to go on holiday over Easter. I'll leave a Fair Isle report with the locum doctor. Expect me early May.'

The next ten minutes are taken up with a discussion of his visit and what it will entail. I'm relieved. We can have an official meeting, and he can answer some questions that aren't easy to discuss due to the crackly phone line.

Saturday is a bright, cold day, but thank goodness it's not raining. I'm feeling more than a little guilty as I wrap up warmly in my hooded jacket and strong boots. I guess not a soul would have objected had I gone to the kirk, but I consider it rude to impose my wishes on centuries of tradition. Anyone seeing me hiking along the cliff tops will surmise that I'm at my favourite hobby.

I find an ideal spot where I'm well hidden. I don't have long to wait until I see the funeral procession emerge from the kirk. Adjusting my binoculars, I watch Reverend Brown, then the eight men – four on each side – dressed in their dark funeral suits. Flashes of white stand out where their shirts peep out from behind black ties.

I shiver and feel goosebumps on my arms as I watch the cortege make its way slowly along the road to the cemetery. I'm glad to have witnessed my very first funeral.

Tears spill as I whisper goodbye.

CHAPTER 27

I love the month of April. After the sadness of March, I can now run to the top of Malcolm's Head, open my arms wide and welcome in new beginnings. Spring is with us, the days are lengthening and the promise of new life is all around. I speak aloud to the mother ewes, and congratulate them on their brand-new baby lambs.

As the daughter of a crofter, and as a midwife, I have a soft spot for sheep, especially at lambing time, and empathise with them if I see them struggling. I've learnt a lot about midwifery from the sheep. Stand back, don't interfere unless necessary, and let nature be your guide.

Edith, the church organist, is organising a choir for Easter. She's invited me to be a member and, because singing is one of my great loves, I agree. My favourite Easter hymn, *All in an April Evening*, is taking pride of place. Edith insists it's got to be perfect so we are busy practising.

'All in an April evening
April airs were abroad
The sheep with their little lambs passed me by on the road ...'

And so on. Every day, I'm living out this hymn.

Men and women are out in the rigs, ploughing and planting, potatoes and oats are already set. Turnip seeds are sown by hand in neat lines. What's more, the weather is kind, with lots of sunny days. It's an idyllic time. Fair Isle is showing off.

Young Stewart, true to his promise, has guided me all over the isle. Birds that have long gone out to sea, or gone to who knows where, are coming back to breed and lay their eggs. We take long sticks with us to ward off the dreaded great skua, or *bonxie*, the Shetland name for these rather ugly-looking aggressive birds that dive-bomb anyone who dares go near their nests. My favourites, the puffins, the Tammie Norries, are starting to make their way back to Fair Isle as well.

'Would you like to come for a spin in my motor boat?' Stewart offers. 'I'll pick a calm day, I know only too well how seasick you can be.'

'Yes, I think that's a good idea. Looking up the cliffs instead of looking down will be an experience.'

We set out on a still, quiet April morning to view Fair Isle from the sea.

Stewart is a competent sailor and I feel safe in his open boat, powered by an outboard motor. The views of the 600-foot cliffs and stacks are magnificent from where I'm sitting and, as Stewart steers his trusty vessel in and out of the various caves and inlets, he points out where ships were wrecked before the lighthouses were built. I'm entranced.

At the entrance to North Haven, Stewart turns off the engine and the boat bobs gently to the rhythm of the waves. The smell of the salt and the sea, the wind through my hair, the burn of the sun on my face, the doorstep-sandwiches and hot flask of tea make this a day to remember. With appetites stimulated by the fresh sea air, we hungrily devour our lunch. Once I've got my breath back, I turn to Stewart, 'The least I can do is help you haul the boat up.'

'It's been a pleasure, Mona. Any excuse to spend a day on the sea. I'm so glad you enjoyed yourself. The bairns will be back in the isle very soon for the Easter holidays. We'll need another dance and a celebration after this long winter.'

'Sounds good to me, Stewart. This time, if I'm not busy, I'll give you a hand with decorating the hall.'

CHAPTER 28

Dr Mainland's pending visit has spurred me on to get the clinic up to standard. With last month's workload, I've neglected it. A peerie devil is whispering in my ear, 'It's a whole month, plenty of time.' But I'm determined to put all procrastination aside and get on with it.

I concentrate on writing administrative reports, ordering medication and equipment, and giving the whole place a once-over. I'm glad I did. I'm feeling a bit smug to have finished already and to have everything so well ordered. And then the phone rings.

Now, who could it be at this time? 10pm. I've lit my wee lamp and I'm thinking longingly of my warm bed. Lifting the phone, I'm already preparing for a call-out.

'Hi there, Mona, it's me, Sheila.'

Of course, my first thought is there must be something wrong at home. 'Oh, hello, is everything okay?'

My peerie sister has never understood my jumping to conclusions. It's my spontaneous personality. She, on the other hand, is logical and thinks things through before she speaks. No wonder she enjoys being a legal secretary.

'Everything is fine,' I hear her laughing. 'Why does du always assume something is wrong, when all I want is a natter and a catch up?'

'Oh, Sheila, du kens me only too well.' I settle down and all thoughts of my cosy bed are forgotten as we laugh and chat and catch up with the home news.

'I'm hoping to come to Fair Isle and have some time wi dee? I had my appendix out last week and I've been signed aff my work for a bit.' Sheila is starting to sound excited.

'Oh, I am sorry about the op,' I say, 'but these days an appendectomy is considered minor surgery. Are you okay?'

'Yes, I'm fine,' Sheila gives a chuckle. 'It's a great excuse for a holiday.'

I can feel the excitement, and hear it in my own voice. 'So, when can I expect dee in?'

'I was thinking about coming for Easter, that's a week away.'

Today's the big 'Sheila' day. I'm feeling happy and excited. I'm glad my house is shining and I've spent a whole day cooking and baking the goodies I know Sheila loves. I'm all ready for my peerie sister. Young Stewart dropped me off at North Haven, then hurried off to attend phone line duties. 'Anne is used to this old pick-up. She'll take you and your sister back home.'

The North Haven is abuzz while we wait for the *Good Shepherd*'s arrival. From where I'm standing, I have a clear view of the harbour mouth and of the *Good Shepherd* as she steams in from the open sea. I see excited school children coming home for the Easter holidays, and there's Anne, Stewart's sister, plus a number of ornithologists and tourists, no doubt as excited as the children at the prospect of viewing rare migrating birds. I'm witnessing a boost to the Fair Isle population, and thinking, maybe more work for me.

I take a step back, watching and enjoying the scene. The Fair Isle primary school children, newly released from their lessons, are whooping and shouting and waving at their brothers, sisters, friends and peers. The incoming Anderson Institute children are making just as much noise, waving at the landlubbers on the quay. I scan the bright faces of the folks on board the *Good Shepherd*, and am amazed at the lack of pale, obviously seasick ones. That's until I spy Sheila.

Oh, no! Knowing exactly how she must be feeling, I run to the gangway to be met by Tommy, for once with a frown and a look of concern on his face. 'She's been very sick and is feeling terrible, you'll have to take care of her.'

Well, well, where did that come from, I wonder? I certainly didn't get that level of attention when I thought I was dying.

Suddenly I realise the jealousy of childhood is surfacing. My beautiful baby sister of the blonde bubble curls and large blue eyes, who has always had everyone entranced, is yet again finding favour over her plain-Jane older sister. For goodness sake, Mona, I scold myself, grow up.

I take Sheila in my arms, noting that she's lost weight. I hear a rasping cough and a sharp intake of breath, as if she's in pain. My big-sister protective emotions kick in and I feel a lump in my throat and detect tears in my eyes.

'I'm so sorry, Mona, I feel awful. All I want to do is get my head down.'

'Say no more. I'll get you home as soon as I have a word with Anne.'

As if on cue, Anne appears at my side. 'I believe I'm giving you a lift. By the look of Sheila, I think we'll waste no time.' And then Anne leans in towards me and confides, 'I feel a bit guilty that I'm feeling bright and breezy. I enjoyed the trip across. Poor Sheila, she wasn't as fortunate, let's get her home.'

Sheila and I squeeze in beside Anne in the front of young Stewart's pick-up. I'm concerned. Sheila is not well, but I keep quiet, forcing a smile. I'll address my concerns once I get home. Anne is sympathetic and I can see she's sized up the situation. Sheila has her eyes closed and her head on my shoulder. Anne of the beautiful singing voice starts to hum, and then very quietly she forms the words of a favourite Shetland ballad. Sheila stirs and says, 'Oh, that is so bonnie, Anne.'

I certainly wasn't expecting this turn of events. Noting her pallor, and listening more carefully to her laboured breathing, it strikes me that Sheila could be really ill. Perhaps her seasickness was masking something more serious?

When we get back to the clinic we help Sheila out of the pick-up and bundle her indoors. Anne watches Sheila collapse onto a kitchen chair. 'I think you should get yourself off to bed, a sleep will do you the world of good.' She lifts her eyebrows, while giving me a knowing look. 'I'm next door, Mona, if you need anything.'

I'm determined not to ask questions until Sheila has had a sleep. Once she's in bed, I bring her a cup of tea and say, 'Now, get that down you and try and sleep if you can.'

I'm rewarded with a watery smile.

I immediately phone mam, asking her to put me in the picture. Mam doesn't sound too concerned. 'She had a bad dose of flu, and then her tummy got very sore, which turned out to be appendicitis.' Mam explains that the operation was a success, but the flu, especially the coughing, got worse and she developed a pain in her side. At first, the surgeon was worried, but after an x-ray and observation he concluded it was just a pulled muscle.

'The surgeon recommended that Sheila go to you for a bit of TLC. Of course, I had no idea what TLC meant. Dad was highly amused and put me right.' We both laugh. I sound a bit hysterical and, to say I'm relieved is an understatement. 'She's got cough medicine and Panadol with her. I know she'll be fine with you.'

When I peep into Sheila's bedroom I'm thrilled to see she's fast asleep and looking comfortable. I have three appointments in the clinic this afternoon. This will take my mind off worrying about Sheila, and talking to mam has reassured me.

After a light supper of fish pie, Sheila tells me she's better. 'The sleep has done me good. I do feel such a fool.' I can see she's angry with herself. 'I'm fine, I really am. It's just this darned pain in my side when I cough. The *Good Shepherd* did me no favours. Sick as a dog I was and, of course, that put extra stress on my side.'

My ears prick up as she goes on. 'A crew member, Tommy, really helped me. He shooed some of the bairns off a bunk – they were just larking about – and he helped me lie down, then he sat with me most of the way. I was past caring what I looked like. I must thank him. He was so very kind.'

Mm, ah ha! Is this love at first sight, or what? I dare not voice my thoughts. I know I would get a smack on my wrist 'for assuming'. I feel myself smiling, though.

On Easter Sunday the bells ring out from the kirk. It's a drizzly day but Sheila and I don't care, we're so happy to be together in our Sunday best. I've roped Sheila in to sing in the choir and, although I say it myself, we sing the old Easter hymns with gusto. Edith is more than pleased. 'I'm happy with you all – sopranos, altos, tenors, and bass – you did me proud.' I will never again sing *All in an April Evening* without thinking about Edith.

Tommy has a strong bass voice. Trust me to notice Sheila giving him an admiring glance.

On our way home from church we stop for a chat with Margaret, Alec's wife. On my rounds, I often stop along Barkland for a cup of tea and try, as far as possible, to avoid Margaret's homebakes. Alas, they are far too yummy and I always succumb. Well, *nearly* always.

Margaret is a cheery, fun-loving woman. 'Pleased to meet you, Sheila. Alec was telling me how poorly you were on the *Good Shepherd*. Hope you're on the mend and feeling better?'

'I'm feeling much better, thank you,' Sheila says, with a smile. 'Mona is looking after me and spoiling me. She's keen I stay until I'm back to normal, so I'm going to do just that.'

'Alec is keen to have a musical evening in the hall next Saturday. Now that the bairns are home and the bird-watchers and tourists are starting to flock to the isle, it seems the right time to have a get-together.'

I tell Margaret to count us in. I'm thinking that this will be a good opportunity for Sheila to get to know the Fair Islanders.

As promised, I help with decorating the village hall. By Saturday night all is set for an evening of song and dance. The whole population of Fair Isle, including the tourists, are invited along. Anyone who can play a musical instrument, and anyone who fancies giving a song, is most welcome. The tables are groaning and the balloons are popping, and we are all having a grand old time, dancing and singing the evening away.

Sheila is still feeling a bit fragile so she sits out the reels and the jigs, but as soon as a waltz is announced, Tommy is across the floor, hand out, and inviting her to dance. The more I watch their faces, the more I'm convinced that a romance is blossoming. This is confirmed when, at the end of the night, Sheila whispers in my ear. 'If you don't mind, Tommy has asked to see me home.'

CHAPTER 29

April continues with mild, changeable weather. My clinic is not busy except for a few minor ailments. I get a call out to see two brothers, home from the Anderson Institute.

'It's chickenpox,' I tell their mam, and hand her a bottle of calamine lotion and a packet of Panadol for the fever. The lads are fed up that their holiday has been ruined. I do sympathise with them, and say, 'I know you're feeling all hot, itchy and miserable, but please try not to scratch.'

I'm hoping that this infectious disease will be contained and not spread throughout the isle.

Apart from that, I feel as if I'm on holiday. Sheila has brightened my life and accompanies me on my house calls. What's more, she has been signed off by the doctor for a full six weeks, so I have her here until the end of May. The romance continues and, in no time at all, word gets out that they're an item. Helen and Lottie are thrilled. They're very fond of Tommy and have taken 'the nurse's sister' to their hearts.

We walk the isle from north to south. The exercise and fresh air has brought the colour back to Sheila's cheeks. The side pain has all but gone, along with the horrible cough. While she's on school holiday, Edith Ann accompanies us. She's a bright girl, full of fun, and the three of us get on like a house on fire. She knows every nook and cranny of her native isle and just when I think I've seen everything possible that I can show Sheila, Edith Ann will have a new surprise up her sleeve.

May. This is my last full month in Fair Isle. Miss Williamson, my superior, phones out of the blue. We have a long conversation and then she finishes by saying, 'I've been keeping my eye on your reports, Nurse Smith. You're very thorough. I like that. Would you be happy to sign up for another year?'

I'm caught off guard. 'Let me give it some thought, and I promise I'll get back to you by the end of May.'

Dr Mainland arrives the first week of May. I meet him at North Haven as he disembarks from the *Good Shepherd*. He's staying at the bird observatory. We've agreed to meet at my clinic every day during his stay.

The first thing he asks me is, 'Are you fond of walking?' When I answer in the affirmative, he seems pleased. 'Great news. I love walking, so no need to bother Stewart Thomson to drive us around unless, of course, the weather is unsuitable.'

This is the first time I've clapped eyes on the man and my first impression is of a mild-mannered fellow in his late forties, with a kind face and a ready smile. I'm used to his voice, and I'm guessing from the cultured tone that he's from Edinburgh. Instinct tells me he is a private person so I don't ask any personal questions.

By 9.00am next morning my small waiting-room is full of people waiting to see Dr Mainland. The very young, the elderly and the less able will be seen when we do house visits. It's a busy week for me and the doctor. Between the clinic and the house visits, time flies past.

It's cold and windy this morning when we set off to visit the North

Lighthouse. It's quite a trek. This lighthouse, like its southerly twin, also houses three families. Mr and Mrs Jones arrived in March with their first baby, ten-week-old Graham. I've been visiting the family regularly since their arrival. Joan and John Jones, young and bewildered by the adorable Graham, keep telling me they 'haven't a clue'. And with no family support they have turned to me, rightly so, for help and advice.

I try my best, but am sorely lacking in health visitor skills. Today, baby Graham has thrush in his mouth and a nasty skin rash. Dr Mainland listens while I voice my opinion. Then he says, 'Nurse is quite right. John, you can drive us back, we'll dispense the medicine and Graham will be right as rain in no time.' I breathe a sigh of relief.

By the middle of May, Dr Mainland has seen all his Fair Isle patients. Tomorrow he's off, back to his practice in Levenwick. I tell myself it's good manners to wave him farewell. With that thought in mind, I'm up early and catch a lift to North Haven. Just before he boards the *Good Shepherd*, he turns to me. 'Are you going to renew your contract and give us another year in Fair Isle?'

'I've been giving it a lot of thought, and no, I'm not. I'm not sure if district nursing is for me, but if I do decide it is, I'll have to do more training.'

His face falls. 'I'm sorry you're not staying, it's of the utmost importance that I can trust and depend on the nurse who looks after Fair Isle. I do wish you well.'

And that is as near as he gets to giving me a compliment.

CHAPTER 30

It's Sheila's last day in Fair Isle and, in two weeks' time, I'll also be on my way back home. It's a fine May morning and we're sitting with our steaming cups of coffee on my kitchen steps.

'Are you sure about Tommy?' I open up the conversation. After all, she's my peerie sister and I do feel responsible for her being in Fair Isle in the first place. From my observations this romance is unfolding very fast − a month − is it really only four weeks since they first set eyes on each other? I take an audible intake of breath and feel my eyes stretching; I've been distracted by Dr Mainland's visit and a full caseload.

'I'm very sure.'

'What does du mean by very sure? It's only been a month.' I'm trying to control the wobble in my voice.

'He's asked me to marry him, and I've said yes.'

I'm dumbfounded. I find my voice, raise it and shout, 'What?' I look at Sheila, really look. Her face is bright and shining and her smile is as wide as my outstretched arms as I hold her close. We're laughing, we're crying and, at last, in a steady tone, I say, 'This is a turn-up for the books. I'm the one who's supposed to be the spontaneous sister.'

'You just know when it's right, and I know for sure this is the right man for me.'

'Well, it's never happened to me,' I reply, with a shake of my head.

'Just you wait, big sister.' Now we're jumping up and down, laughing. Caddy, my sheep friend, gives a quizzical stare and then goes on grazing her patch of lawn.

Tommy is coming for tea. It's time to celebrate. We spend the afternoon baking a Victoria sandwich and some chocolate biscuits.

'Tommy, du's a dark horse,' I tell him, as we settle down for Sheila's farewell tea.

'I couldn't believe my luck when she consented to marry me. I can still hardly believe it. Mum and dad know, but before we can broadcast the news I'll need to come to Whiteness and spör your dad for Sheila's hand.'

I'm tickled pink at this old-fashioned courtesy and tell Tommy I couldn't wish for a better brother-in-law.

CHAPTER 31

Miss Williamson's call came the last day of May. 'Before you say anything, Nurse Smith, I've had a word with Dr Mainland and he tells me that you're not renewing your Fair Isle contract. He also said that you might consider district nursing.'

'Yes, that's right. I might consider it, but I'm still not sure as it means extra training.'

Miss Williamson then proposes an option for me. Shetland only has one fully-trained health visitor and there is a need for more. 'The academic year starts in August at Queen Margaret's University, Edinburgh. If you're up for it, you can apply. Our local authority will pay your salary while you train and, what's more, will pay for driving lessons. We can't have a Queen's district nurse unable to drive. You will, of course, have to give us back two years post-training.'

I tell Miss Williamson this is a lot to take in and I'll need to give it thought. Once I'm back in Shetland, in the middle of June, I'll give her my decision.

Then I put my future away and focus on my last two weeks in Fair Isle. I have time to reflect on my year spent in this beautiful, wild and wonderful isle and I ask myself what I've learned, if anything. What is it that I'll take away with me?

Nursing: what is it about, I ask myself? The theory is important. All-important too is meticulous record-keeping. On-going education and keeping up to date with evidence-based treatment and the continuous striving for excellence. Yes, but that's the easy part. We nurses can all learn that. There is something more, isn't there? Something more difficult to put your finger on. What is it?

I sit for hours brooding. It comes to me in bite-sized answers. It's about experience. I'm still young. I'm just starting out on my nursing journey. But after this year in Fair Isle I'm beginning to trust myself. More and more I find myself disregarding the rule book. I no longer rely on guidelines to connect situations. I've had to rely on myself, to trust my gut reaction, and then to stop and think logically.

I've learned, too, that patients trust me. A bed bath, an injection, the suturing of a wound, a new treatment – all these are taken for granted. It's what I say, and how I make my patients feel that's the all-important factor. Can this be learnt? If I'm ever in a position to teach junior nurses, I'll try.

I visit each house and say my final goodbye. I'm getting good at hiding my feelings and swallowing down my tears. I will never forget how the Fair Isle folk made me feel. My time with them has changed me forever. I have matured and grown in my belief in myself. I have learnt so much – about myself and my abilities certainly, but also about friendship, about community, about kindness. These are the gifts they have given me, and which I will carry with me for the rest of my life.

I board the *Good Shepherd* and dismiss all thoughts of seasickness; it's a calm day. I must get home now and ask dad what he thinks about Miss Williamson's proposal.

A MIDWIFE
IN AFRICA

If you enjoyed this memoir there's another one in the offing – A Midwife in Africa is coming out in 2023.

FAIR ISLE
'THEN'

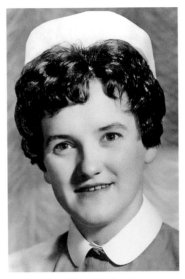

Mona, 1960s.

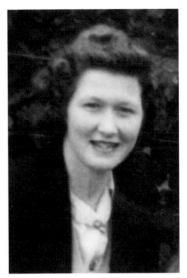

Annie Thomson, photo courtesy
of Anne Sinclair.

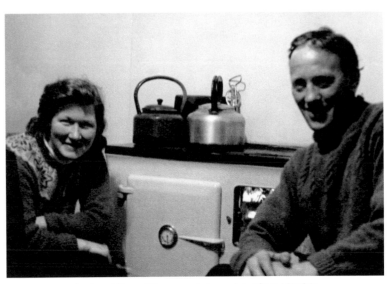

Annie and Stewart Thomson, photo courtesy of Anne Sinclair.

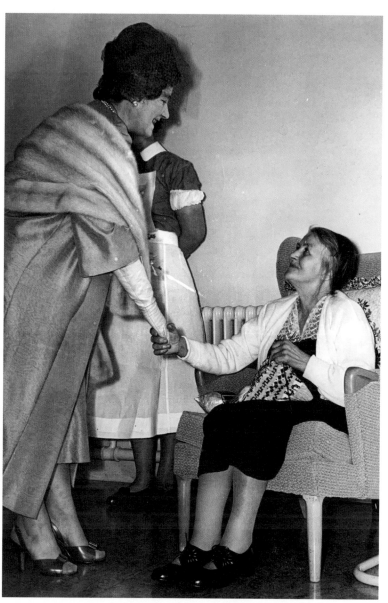

The Queen Mother visiting Gilbert Bain Hospital, meeting Maggie.
Photo courtesy of Dennis Coutts.

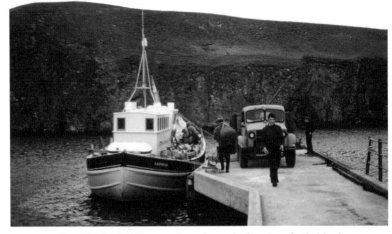

'Good Shepherd II'. The men pictured are unloading stores for the island and it is believed that the Queen and Prince Philip were transported on the back of the same truck when they visited Fair Isle in the 1960s.

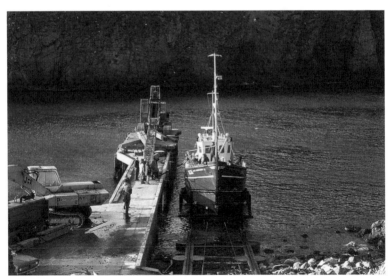

North Haven, 'Good Shepherd III'.

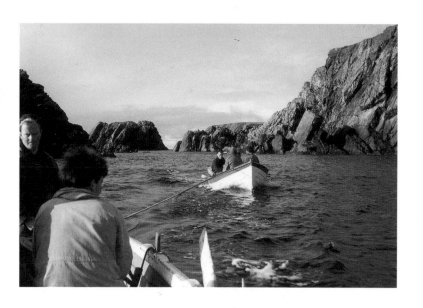

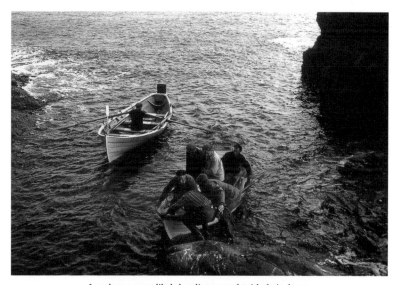

Local men, most likely heading to work with their sheep.

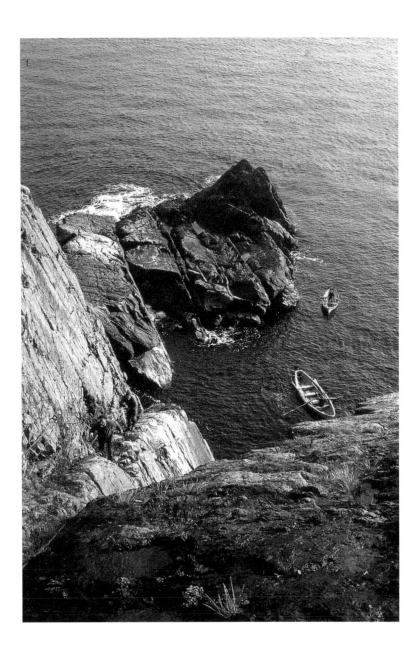

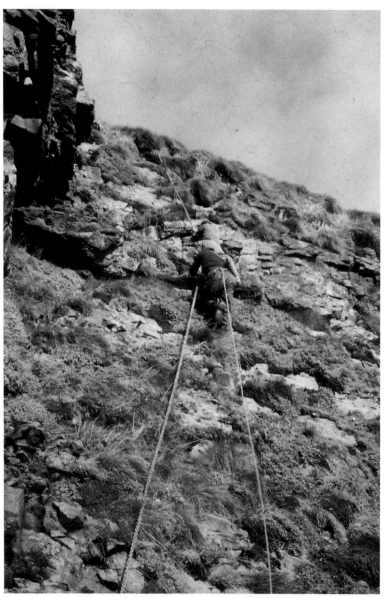

Local men climbing up a steep cliff face.

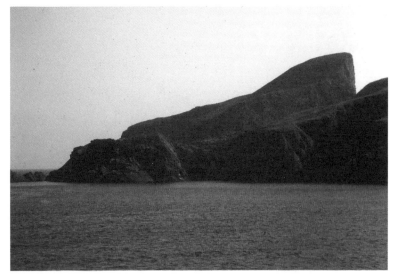

Sheep Rock.

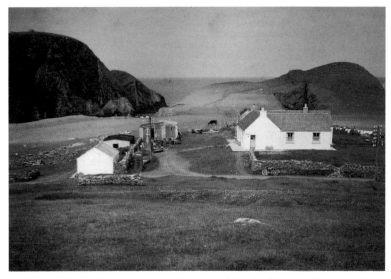

Stewart and Annie Thomson's house with the clinic behind and the post office to the left.

FAIR ISLE
'NOW'

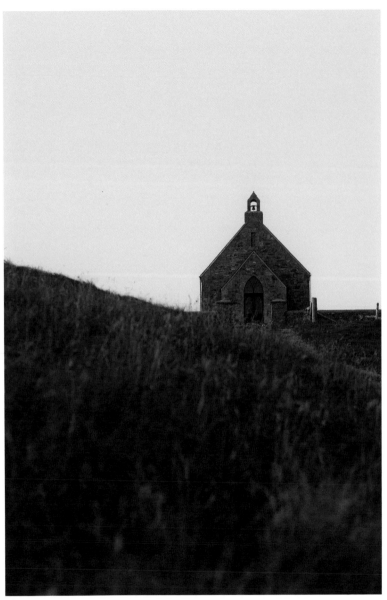
The Methodist Chapel.

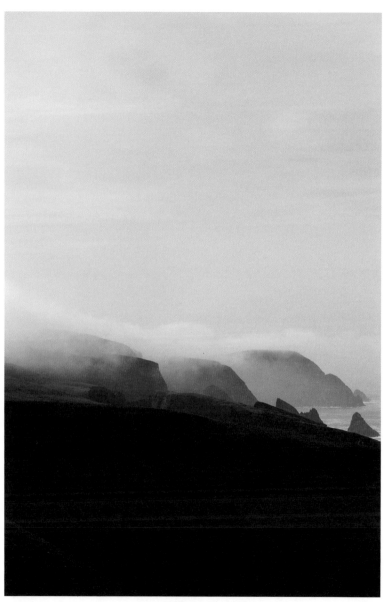
Fair Isle cliffs shrouded in mist.

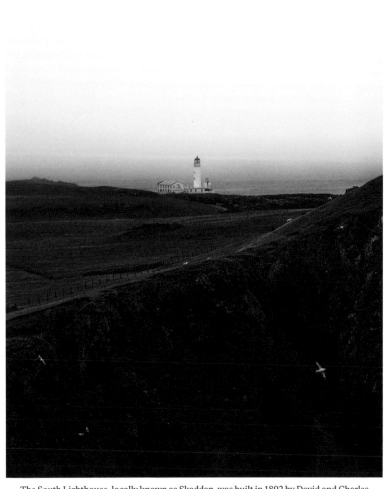

The South Lighthouse, locally known as Skaddan, was built in 1892 by David and Charles Stevenson and it was the last Scottish manned lighthouse to be automated.

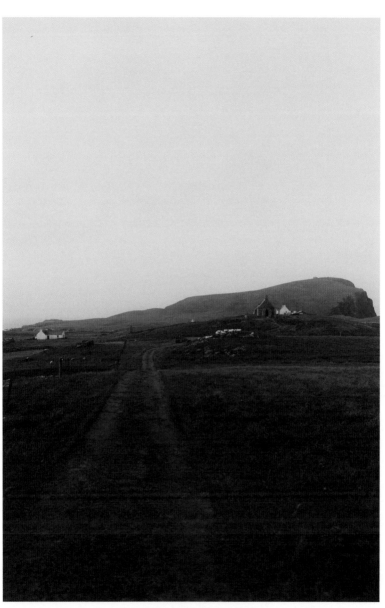

The view towards Malcolm's Head.

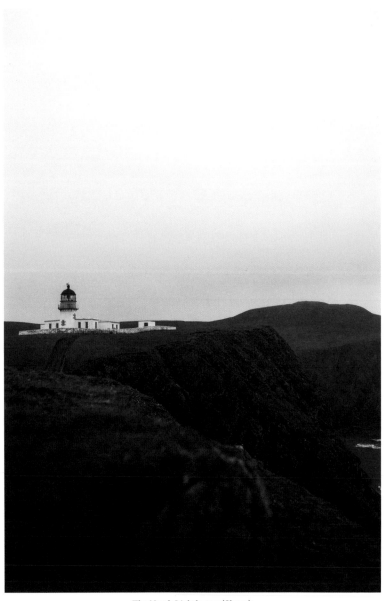

The North Lighthouse (Skroo).

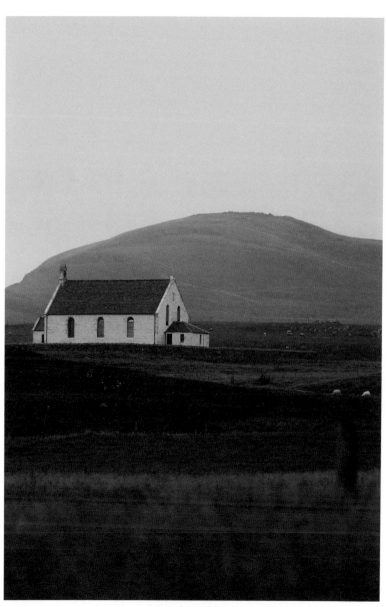

Church of Scotland Kirk.

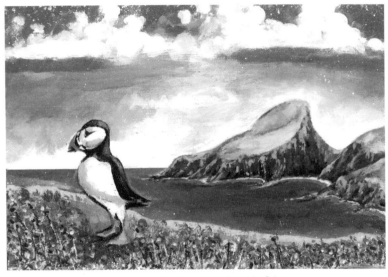

A Fair Isle inspired painting by Sven McAlpine.